'C'

a story for
Couples
coming and going

From Chapter 2:
"Do you prefer Brillo or S.O.S?"
—"My preference is 'maid'."
(Reader: "I would buy that book!")
—More Reader comments on back cover.

Ted and Sharon,
Many thanks for very enjoyable
visits.
Coming or going, wherever the Road
leads, Rejoice.

Richard E. Schirgoethe

'C'

a story for
Couples
coming and going

RES
Richard E. Schingoethe

AuthorHouse
Bloomington, IN

Image Credits:
Cover   ©iStockphoto.com/jhorrocks
Chapter 1   ©iStockphoto.com/Yuri_Arcurs
Chapter 2   ©iStockphoto.com/Klubovy
Chapter 3   ©iStockphoto.com/mocker_bat
Chapter 4   ©iStockphoto.com/sjlocke
Chapter 5   ©iStockphoto.com/Lokibaho
Chapter 6   ©iStockphoto.com/Pidjoe
Chapter 7   ©iStockphoto.com/EyeJoy

ISBN: 978-1-4490-1044-7 (hc)
       978-1-4490-1045-4 (sc)

LCCN: 2009907354

Published by
AuthorHouse
1663 Liberty Dr. Suite 200
Bloomington, IN 47403
Visit *www.authorhouse.com* for additional information.

First published by AuthorHouse 8/7/2009

Printed in the United States of America

For would-be Couples everywhere.
Past and current Couples, too.

Dedicated to the Partner
who inspires and believes in me
as no one else ever has
or, I suspect,
ever will.

<RES>

'C'

A story for

Couples

coming and going

*"Many times I thought I couldn't live with you.
And many times I know I can't live without you."*

CONTENTS

1.   Finding your 'C'-mate   *"Happiness sometimes arrives unexpected ..."*

2.   Getting to know you   *"Do you prefer Brillo® or SOS®?"*
    "My preference is 'maid'!"

3.   Merging   *"Will you marry me?"*
    "I would love to."

4.   Daily Doses   *"I just called to say I'm thinking about you and I love you and I miss you."*

5.   2nd-Thinking   When occasional 'hiccups' raise 'red flags.'

6.   Un-Coupling   She drove 223 miles, just to say 'Good-by.'

7.   Post-Couple Coupling   *"... many times I know I can't live without you."*

*"Many times I thought
I couldn't live with you.*

*"And many times I know
I can't live without you."*

It's a dilemma faced by many of us in love and relationships. And numerous "how to" books (including tomes by umpteen PhDs) dispense advice on these subjects.

Now comes "'C': a story for Couples coming and going" — filled with anecdotes and observations, wisdom and wit, by a writer who has simply lived it … in ways that frequently mirror our own.

With a unique, refreshing blend of narrative, musical lyrics and quotable quotes, 'C' takes us on a journey through the phases of Coupling … from "Finding your 'C'-Mate," to "Un-Coupling" and even "Post-Couple Coupling."

'C' is, in truth, a story — a story that draws on the author's life 'n times to give us a highly perceptive view of what happens at various stages in relationships, while offering actionable ideas that help make Coupling more fun.

Sometimes funny, heartwarming or even heartbreaking, 'C' makes no pretenses about being more than its title implies.

Whatever your age or relationship stage, chances are 'C' can help make your Couple-times more meaningful, more enjoyable.

Perhaps because, in many ways, 'C' is every reader's story, too.

Author's Note

Being a Couple is, in some ways, rather simple: put two people together and — ka-boom! — you have a Couple.

No matter how much (or little) a Couple has in common, however, when two forces converge, a multitude of factors — many of which you "can't quite put your finger on," can create …

"Speed bumps on the Highway to Forever."

Speed bumps can rise up among Couple-seeking Singles as well as current Couples … at any age or stage. They can enhance or aggravate — or ultimately detour the entire relationship.

I've "been there, done that" on virtually all fronts in more than a few Couplings and, it seems to me …

We could all use a little help — maybe the kind provided in 'C'.

Drawn from my past and several special colleagues … the following pages offer anecdotes and observations, philosophical "nuggets," plus tips & tidbits, "takeaway" ideas, and a few questions to ponder.

Whether you're a 20-something, a mid-lifer or retirement age … currently Coupling, un-Coupling or at stages in-between …

… I hope 'C' will help smooth-out "speed bumps" that you may encounter, reawaken warm memories, and make your Couple-times more meaningful — just as writing this, has made mine.

<RES>
res@canterburylane.com

3

Chapter 1

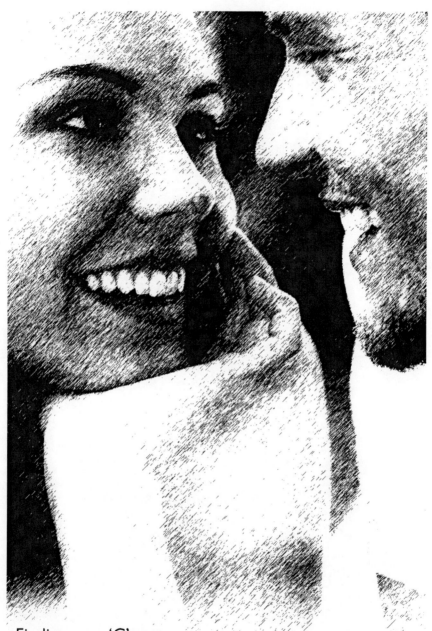

Finding your 'C'-mate

"Happiness sometimes
arrives unexpected …"

"Happiness sometimes

arrives unexpected ..."

... Like you
and me and the life we've elected.

Could this be the 'We' in our
partnership quest?

Our hearts speak as one
and the answer is 'Yes.'

" ... a happiness surprise

woven into the fabric

of our daily lives."

<u>You never know ...</u>

... where, when or how your 'C'-mate may arrive. For me, it's ranged all over the lot.

There was the flight attendant. Yep, we met on a plane.

The sales rep ... met at a conference.

A teacher whose class starred in a video for a client.

The "blind date" whose girlfriend's boyfriend gave me her number and suggested I call. (I did.)

The PR exec, while working on joint-client projects.

The school teacher who "got me over a barrel." (I can explain; but not here, now.)

A former coworker, when our paths later crossed.

A visitor from out of town, introduced by mutual friends.

And — oh, yeah ... a woman I "coached" through the trauma of divorce; then ignored the Coaches Manual where it says "don't get involved."

From *where* your 'C'-mate arrives, however, is of little import. What matters is that he or she does. (Besides, this isn't a how-to book on finding dates, although we will touch on some options.)

What do you look for? How can you tell?

Good questions. With answers as varied as each person who asks — multiplied by every candidate you find.

Nevertheless, when trying to decide if that person you started seeing is Mr. or Ms. Right, here are a few clues ...

Where ...

.. does one start
in matters of the heart?

Maybe with eyes
that see you as you.
Ears eager to hear
daily things that you do.

Words that can comfort,
inform and inspire.
Lips willing to waken
or await your desire.

Fingers that touch you
with kindness and care.
Soft, quiet music;
a cheek 'gainst your hair.

Arms that can cradle
and also turn loose.
Warm smiles and laughter
that need no excuse ...

Where'er you begin,
wherever you start,
you'll find they entwine
in matters of the heart.

And I pray you will find
that mine fill your needs.

Will you open your heart?
Dare I hope where it leads?

© RES²

'Opposites attract' ...

... so the saying goes. Often, it's true. And exciting, too!

Suddenly you're seeing and doing new things, meeting new people who are more interesting (or at least different) than the crowd you're used to.

While "opposites" may attract, can such relationships last? Common ground typically provides a more solid foundation.

The answer is ... "Yes" and "No." (No surprise here.)

I've seen "city slickers" and country folks (my own parents, for instance) become close partners for life. You probably can point to many examples, too. However ...

Matching lifestyles <u>can</u> help you team-up with ease.

One woman I know encountered a man who mirrored in many ways the life she was used to and, frankly, liked. He had everything on her list:

Megabucks ... superb golfer ... gourmet cook. He was also a DIY fix-it whiz around the house. And, I presume, a reasonably decent lover. Who could ask for more?

Well ... maybe both parties.

Surface similarities cement nothing "for keeps." The adhesive that brings (and holds) a Couple together comes from a far deeper, inner source.

Sometimes you can also detect hints regarding Mr. or Ms. Right from "outside" sources ...

Pets, believe it or not ...

... could provide a clue. And I don't mean "take your 'Berner' to the dog park" and find someone with a similar canine companion.

Maybe it's my Midwestern farm upbringing, but I have a very high regard for animal intelligence and instincts. In particular, dogs.

> _"Never trust a man that_
> _a dog doesn't like."_

> _"Or a woman_
> _who doesn't like dogs."_

Although to my knowledge there is no documentation to support such statements, I have no qualms making them.

Note the word "trust." ... A crucial clue when deciding with whom you want to be. It's a fitting companion for another suggestion:

Go with your gut. (Even if you might get kicked in it.)

Forget "ideal mate — matching lifestyles" criteria, and "plusses vs. minuses" lists.

If it feels right to you, it's the right thing to do.

Of course, my own Couples track record makes it easy to question such wisdom.

But, hey — I've no regrets. It's been one heckuva ride.

net-escape

You sent me to your site
— banished me
to *the net.*

Now the cursor crawls
carrying me down
past dim-lit words
deep into the dark
mine-shaft
night

suddenly,
exploding arms reach,
welcome me in …
warm, moving, bright
slivers of light
electric
touch …

'Disposable Society'
aka Internet ...

On-line matchmaking, in some ways, offers many advantages over visiting local bars and clubs or other hangouts in order to meet someone.

On the other hand, if you haven't yet learned from your own experience, watching a few movies (such as "Must Love Dogs") will quickly alert you to the outright lies and deceit running rampant throughout the cyberspace dating scene.

Disposable? Indeed.

That said, such awareness can equip you with the take-it-with-a-grain-of-salt attitude to cope with reality bytes whenever actual contact occurs.

What's more, two can play the game (and millions do). So you could, if you choose, have a bit of fun fooling folks yourself.

And hopefully, when you and your potential 'C'-mate meet for real, your senses of humor will prevail.

Finding a 'C'-mate ...

... certainly doesn't require a cyberspace jump-start. The best way to get things going, perhaps, is to not try so hard.

"Do less looking — more enjoying."

Enjoy the life you lead. What you do, where you are, the people and activities around you. An upbeat outlook clarifies your view of anything & anyone you see. More importantly, you'll look and act your best. And letting "the real you" show through, dramatically improves your chances of someone else ... finding you.

"Happiness sometimes
arrives unexpected ..."

Far away or close to home? Either or both, of course. One man I know was blown away by a woman he met in a bar. In Puerto Rico. While vacationing with buddies after the island wedding they were to attend ... was called off.

Another found his 'C'-mate in the cast of a rock-dance revue produced by the theatre company of which he was a member.

As it turns out, the "Puerto Rico Connection" lived in New Jersey and he lived in Chicago. Which made her "G-U" (Geographically Undesirable). Don't let such "speed bumps" deter you or detour your relationship, however.

14

From afar: real mail, real voices

The difficulties of maintaining (much less building) a long-distance relationship are many, and well documented.

Not to worry. The idea is to get to a point where you truly want to be together. Then you'll find a way.

> "Where
> did you say you live?"

> "Since you,
> I've been living on
> 'Cloud 9' ..."

Of course, computers offer fast, inexpensive and instantly received messaging. Nevertheless, e-missiles instantly sent, can be just as instantly deleted. ("Disposable Society" ... remember?)

And, as a Public Relations exec once wrote: "Never confuse e-mail with communicating."

She's so right.

It's tough to top a real-mail letter. Even better, a beautifully penned, handwritten note.

(A Missile in the Mail)

*"I am thinking of your fabulously
awesome eyes,"*

she wrote.

*"Those beautiful droplets of blue ice.
Or are they puddles of glistening
aquamarine Mediterranean?*

*"Either way, they reflect so much
of what they see.
Those all-knowing, all seeing,
understanding eyes
of yours ... pools of knowledge,
brimming with tenderness,
love and concern.*

*"The best thing
is when your beautiful eyes
look into mine."*

Wow. And not so incidentally, you could send a
note like this to someone living next door, too!

16

And if it's real-time ...

... give-and-take long distance communication you want, go with the telephone.

I have, time and again. From my first fianceé to the last, telephones have provided the conduit connecting our words, hearts and minds.

> _"You sound wonderful,"_
> _she said_
> _"... that husky, smoky_
> _voice of yours ..."_

The telephone's a great tool with which to generate and share ideas and excitement about almost anything. You can even (trust me on this) stoke passion fires to incredible intensity.

And, even more frequently, over long- (or short-) distance lines, you can experience some of life's most tender, memorable moments ...

You drifted into dreamland ...

... even as I spoke
   (softly, of course)
   into the phone.

And I don't know if you heard me
say that
   the one (and maybe only)
"reassurance"
   I can give you
is that
   I care for you.

I am here for you
     no matter where,
   geographically,
we may be.

Silence says
that peaceful rest
has wrapped its arms around you

just as I, once more,
     cradle you in my mind,
   hold you in my heart.

No need for you to wake
and "listen" to me speak.

A thousand miles
could be a million;

It matters not,
when someone feels
   as I do about you.
Pleasant dreams ...

"Can't see the forest ...

... for the trees," the saying goes. Well, sometimes the opposite is true:

You can be looking so far and so hard at the overall forest, that you don't see the trees ... right under your nose.

Several cases-in-point come to mind from my 'C'-mate experience — some going back to elementary school days, or involving former coworkers who were nothing-but that until we discovered far more in each other. (A cautionary note: the old adage "Don't sleep where you work" still rings true; it could prevent multiple problems.)

Point is: you need not necessarily look too far.

Next door

We grew up next-door neighbors.
You had your friends. I had mine.
   We'd seldom talk.
   Never took a walk,
which suited me just fine.

But now I'm
   Hot for your body!
   Love to touch your skin.
   Come to my arms,
   with newfound charms.
Let's love 'til who-knows-when!

Can't explain why it happened.
Each of us, out on our own.
   But suddenly
   as you brushed past me
I noticed how you've grown!

And I am
   Hot for your body!
   Love to touch your skin.
   Come to my arms,
   with newfound charms.
Let's love 'til who-knows-when!

Best of all, we both feel it.

Seems too good to be true

    that we'll find more

    lovin' next door

than either of us knew!

Oh, I'm so

    Hot for your body!

    Love to touch your skin.

    Come to my arms,

    with newfound charms.

Let's love 'til who-knows-when!

"I remember the first time" ...

Doesn't everyone? Fondly, I hope.

Perhaps my most memorable "first time in bed" occurred
during the wee small hours when, standing bedside, I pulled up
the covers, tucked-in my 'C'-mate and stepped away to sleep
elsewhere.

Suddenly her hand was in mine, gently pulling me back. "No ...
It's OK." She drew me closer and I whispered, "Are you sure
...?" It took a few moments for her to convince me that she was.
Tentatively, I slid under the covers, wrapped my arms around
her and ...

... We fell asleep, almost instantly, resting peacefully, blissfully —
better than I had in years (if ever). Then for the first time, we
discovered the wonder of waking up to each other's smiling eyes.

> *"You're my part-time lover,*
> *full-time Love."*

Point is: *Take care not to confuse* sexual attraction with "love"
(whatever that means; I suspect it's a uniquely individual or, if you
will, Couple thing).

More than that, I sincerely hope sexual <u>satisfaction</u> will play a
role in your 'C'-mate relationship. There is a world of difference
between passionate sexual intercourse and a truly gratifying
experience.

22

Many attributes ...

... beliefs and attitudes can draw you toward potential partners. Mannerisms, too — some of which can also be off-putting.

Which brings me to sort of an "issue" with me ... one that probably won't make one iota of difference to most people, or impact relationships. Nevertheless ...

Over the years, one question has repeatedly come to mind — actually, it's been <u>brought</u> to my mind by various women I've known.

To wit:

why 'me'?

Why do so many women
in relationships with men
adopt the moniker
                    "me"?

In phone conversations
        "Hi, it's me."
In letters and e-mails
            "See you soon"
        "Take care"
    "Love"…
"Me" " Me" "Me"

…as if her given name
weren't special enough
or important enough
                    to you
to merit
    recognition and use.

Or maybe each feels she is
the only person in your life
        who qualifies
for that pronoun
(thus making her more than
    just another
    anonymous "me").

Perhaps she considers "me"
    a term of endearment
or, more than that, a test:
        Can you name
        the real "me"?
(Contestant number three?)

Why hide?
…when you've been given
                    so much more?
    (At least so it is with those
        I've loved and known.)

See them…say them…

Arielle and Adrianne
Jo Ann and Joanne
Susan and Suzanne...

Kathryn and Cathleen,
Sarah, Sara Jean
Sharon and Darlene
Helen and Marlene...

Karnilla and Priscilla,
Deborah, Debra,
Darcy, Deanna,
Pamela, Melissa...

Ella, Nancy, Peggy,
Janet and Renee;
Lina, Tina, Diane,
Donna Rae and Mary Kay...

Heather and Esther,
Tamara, Evelyn;
Lori and Laura,
Caroline, Carolyn...

Merrida Sue, Mary Lou,
Kimberly, Natalie,
Julie, Leslie and Judy...

"What's in a name?"
the age-old question goes
             or
"what *is* a name?"
The answer's the same
    in the vision I see
embracing far more than "me."

It's a special term for You
            and the first
    sight or sound
each time you write or speak
    that makes you
    so special

        to me.

Music and dancing ...

... offer ice-breaking opportunities, whether you're with a 'C'-mate or looking to hook-up.

Not-so-incidentally, on the dance floor you can initiate physical contact and express body language that can further enhance verbal communication. In short — a lot of good stuff happens here.

I've enjoyed more than a few major indoor and outdoor concerts and related events — exciting, impressive performances that make both parties feel special. And give you special memories to take with you, long-term.

A proliferation of nearby neighborhood and community venues, however, offer daily (perhaps "nightly" is more correct) getaway opportunities — usually for the price of a few drinks.

Here you can "lose yourself" with a partner. And that, in my experience, can be a very good thing.

Season of Now

Your silk-smooth locks
   caress my cheek
      and we move as one
         through the Blues band's
"Midnight Lovers' Set."

The calendar and the chill night air
say it's Autumn, going on Winter.

But we have more.
Right here. Right now.

There's Summer sunshine
   in your smile,
a Springtime sparkle
   in your laugh,
a warm and gentle breeze
   in your soft words
       and a hint of
… (who knows?) to come.

Tonight we find a bright new day.

Tomorrow …?
Don't ask.
Don't disrupt
   the music of the moment,
the magic of now.

You see, now is where we live,
not merely when.

And as each "now" arrives, flows
through and moves on …

   for us, it is

a Season unending.

The greatest love ...

... of my life brings a blend of many Couple-making aspects touched upon so far.

Music and dancing play big roles with Us.

She doesn't make "me" her moniker. She calls me by name — and loves to hear me speak hers.

She's also someone I've known since childhood.

We stayed in touch over the years (telephone, real-mail and, yes, even e-mail) while living in different states and raising separate families. From family crises (serious illnesses, major surgeries, parents' passing) through wedding celebrations and the like, we have supported and "been there for" each other.

Then we found each other as a Couple quite suddenly and unexpectedly when divorce (which I experienced some years ago) became a reality in her life, too.

At the time, she lived hundreds of miles away.

While our ultimate Couple-ship may not extend to the nth degree, we have found an extraordinary kinship that few (if any) other Couples enjoy.

To me, when seeking your 'C'-mate for life, the message is simple:

Follow your Heart.

You will find the Kindred Spirit who enriches your Soul.

Chapter 2

Getting to know you

"Do you prefer Brillo® or SOS®?"

"My preference is 'maid'!"

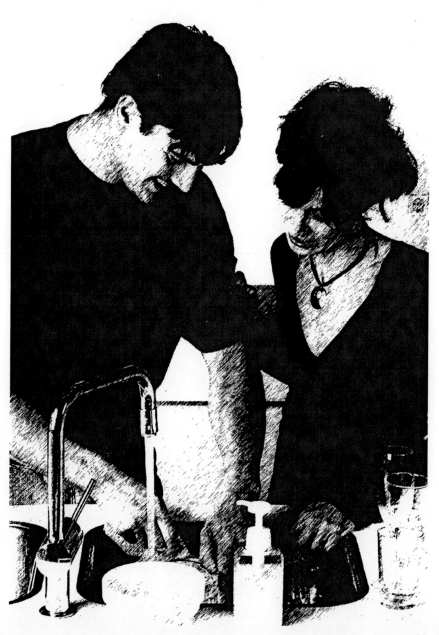

We both laughed out loud

… and, of course, agreed that a maid or other household assistance would be more to our liking.

With this anecdote, however, comes a bigger thought:

If thinking beyond dates & nightlife scares the daylights out of you, fear not.

Everyday chores and routine things need not be a "necessary evil." All work and no play, of course, doesn't sound too exciting. So when there is housework 'n all to do, find ways to have fun with it, too.

Go ahead — jump in with both feet. Somehow, you'll muddle through. And you and your partner will quickly discover so much more in each (and both) of you.

As a 'C'-mate of mine put it:

"Love isn't a word. It's an action."

happy daze

It's the day-to-day
times we share
— things we do
that say "I care."

Maybe it's a glance,
a touch, a kiss …
Or hands helping
you to wash a dish.

Helping clasp/unclasp
    a bracelet,
or zip-up a top.
Or an honest
"You look great!"
    even when
you think you're not.

Bringing me coffee
    in the morning,
bringing your bedside
    water glass at night.
Holding doors open,
and taking care of insects
that give you fright …

There are oh-so many things
        with me 'n you.
Even saying "I love you"
    once more reveals
that, in truth, we do.

So revel in the wonder
        of "happy daze."
It makes for happy days.
And also happy nights.

Despite love-at-first-sight

scenarios, finding someone to date (even steadily) does not mean you've found a 'C'-mate. No way. Not yet.

It takes more than that — and, yes, more than sex — to qualify for real.

For openers, "sight" involves only one of the senses. There's no question, of course, that physical attraction makes up much of that "first impression." Fashionable attire can convey surface messages, too.

Once you meet 'n greet and start to talk — backgrounds, jobs, current events, likes and dislikes — topics galore, you start discovering attitudes and ideas, maybe also hopes and dreams … You get a closer, fuller, deeper look (pun intended) at the person you see.

Now, mentally and emotionally, you'll start to feel drawn toward — or pushed away.

If it's the former and the two of you continue, the process takes you to many more levels, different venues … and routinely involves all of your "human senses" and more.

As for the eyes … well … sometimes, far-from-fancy "non-evening" attire can inspire love at first sight, too.

They were soft, white ...

... terry cloth shorts. Hot-pants length. Long ago, I wore them when playing tennis. I must say they look much better on her — conforming to her curves, beautifully.

She teamed them with a faded, often-worn, often-washed (yes, "off-white") T-shirt emblazoned with the logo of my university _alma mater._

Thus was born her outfit for cleaning around the house. And for de-furring my cats. (Hadn't seen anyone do that before and — wow! — was she good!) Never saw so much cat hair in my life. A mountain of fur-ball fodder.

They hated it. And loved her for doing it.

Clothing-and-cat specifics aside,

... what matters most between you two, isn't what you wear — but rather, what you do.

A myriad of day-to-day home life, social life and special events await exploration, participation ... to advance the Couple of You.

All it takes is your willingness to try.

The Great
Grapefruit Challenge

Is it quicker to cut a grapefruit crossways, slice each bite-size
section and sprinkle on a little sugar …?

… Or to peel it entirely, pull apart full-slice halves and pull off the
inner "skin" — leaving slices ready to eat?

I recall debating this with a 'C'-mate via long-distance phone,
while preparing grapefruits in our respective homes.

We vowed to sometime compete face-to-face, with a Stopwatch
to document preparation times.

We never actually did it. But the Challenge certainly helped us
connect as a Couple.

Everyone wins.

Friends 'n Family ...

... can provide new insights and/or add dimensions to those you already have regarding your 'C'-mate as you meet, socialize or otherwise associate with them.

This works both ways, from both sides. His or her friends and family may fill you in on skills, accomplishments, interests and events ... perhaps revealing more things that you have in common, or opening new avenues for the two of you to pursue together. And vice versa — your friends & family filling in your 'C'-mate on parts of your life to-date.

And feedback from both sides will keep the ball rolling.

Even some of those "embarrassing" childhood or other "family secrets," at this age & stage of your lives, may be more likely to trigger smiles and warm feelings ... and/or reveal positive characteristics or traits that you will find endearing.

> Of course, each of you will (to some degree, at least) be "under the microscope" while all of this is going on.

Movies have been made about meeting the family of girlfriends/ boyfriends, fiancées 'n such. For the most part, they're "romantic comedies," with lots of laughs stemming from (yes) real-life attitudes and situations.

And to be sure, the prospect can be a bit frightening.

Anything sound familiar?

_"He's been hurt
so often ..."_

"It's too soon (since
break-up, divorce, whatever). She
needs time ..."

_"What do they have in
common? He's 'country,' and she's
'Country Club' ..."_

_"... on the rebound; just
looking for someone
to fill a gap ..."_

_"... don't know what
she (he) sees in
him (her)."_

_"She's only after
his money."_

_"... not ready
for a 'permanent'
relationship ..."_

<u>Don't be surprised ...</u>

... if family members have reservations about you and your 'C'-mate. For that matter, friends and even business associates may voice concerns, too.

For example, if either or both of you have accumulated wealth to any significant degree (inheritance, insurance benefits, divorce settlement ...) relatives may be joined by "financial planners" injecting warnings into the mix, ostensibly in the interest of protecting client assets.

"They love me and are concerned about me," insisted one woman I know, as questions and objections continued to mount from various sources. I don't doubt her for a minute.

> And prenuptial agreements are a frequent,
> obvious way to ease financial concerns.

Not so easily resolved are more-personal attitudes and issues that may arise within your or your 'C'-mate's families.

These could run the gamut from not liking "the way she does her hair" or aversion to his aftershave, to religious issues or political leanings.

If your 'C'-mate has alerted you to "lightning rod" topics, you may want to avoid them.

On the other hand, I sometimes enjoy pushing "hot buttons" and seeing where the sparks fly. It's a good way to learn a lot, quickly. And it sure can liven up an evening!

Fan-atical

She stepped into his brother's home for the first time and immediately found her carefully coiffed hair mussed and her thoughtfully chosen, meticulously tailored outfit hidden under an ill-fitting jersey emblazoned with the local sports team's logo.

It was "game day."

Surrounded by cheering "fans" whom she'd never met before, she smiled and graciously acknowledged being welcomed as "one of us."

Truth be known, she doesn't much give a rip for football.

If you and your 'C'-mate haven't yet been in situations like this, chances are (sooner or later) you will be. Simple tip:

It never hurts to be a good sport.

"Never listen to the reviewers."

Doing things to please your partner and to "fit in" with friends & family — or business associates — is both commendable and likely to generate positive vibes. Including vibes coming from within you.

The only (obvious) caution is to avoid trying too hard. Over-reaching will almost certainly be detected, and those you're trying to impress will probably be put off.

In short, don't try to be something or someone you're not. Remember:

> Many a movie or play has been panned by "experts," only to break box-office records.

Just be yourself — let the real "you" show through.

If other people can't handle that, it's their problem. Sure, you'll want to pay attention to what they say, think, how they respond.

The ultimate response is yours. And it must be one (as the saying goes) that you can live with.

Part of the process is to assess family & friends' attitudes and issues which you observed — positive as well as negative — with your 'C'-mate … and see how they impact your views (if at all), individually and as a Couple.

You'll do things ...

... that you've done before — but never before, together.

Like go to church (or a synagogue, cathedral, whatever). In one case I recall, my 'C'-mate and I had been "raised" in the same religion, had attended mutual-family weddings and such over the years.

Our first church service as a Couple (honest-to-God, no pun intended) was on ... "Passion Sunday."

Then we went to brunch at a lovely riverside restaurant.

Far less ethereal are things you do that (until now, at least) you don't particularly enjoy.

For example, I'm not much of a "shopper"; wandering around malls and big stores isn't my thing. But I paid my first visit to IKEA with a 'C'-mate in search of bed linens for her daughters, material to line cupboard shelves and more.

It was fun. And I discovered "cart-scalators" — escalators that take shopping carts from floor to floor. What a hoot.

And she, who fears heights, rode the Ferris Wheel with me at a county fair one sunny afternoon. She still hated being so high … but smiled all the way. I love her for it, still today.

In the process, all of this touches deeper feelings, too.

You may even sense an "ethereal impact" — an occurrence that makes you think "maybe, just maybe" the two of you share a wavelength that transcends anything on earth …

(A Missile in the Mail)

<u>'I felt you stir ...'</u>

"From across the miles

... I felt you stir.

I looked at the clock;
it was 3:40 a.m.

I hoped that you
were still in bed
so that your warm,
firm body could
cradle me again ...

... from across the miles."

<u>"Morning person" vs. "Evening" …</u>

I often arose in the wee small hours, when she might just be going to bed. — Not usually when we were together, mind you; but when we were hundreds of miles apart, each of us dealing with unique schedule demands.

Could this morning/evening difference derail your relationship in a merged-Couple setting?

With a little thought and effort, the two of you can find comfortable middle ground.

And even on those occasions when individual work or other demands arise, there are ways to make it work for you … special things that you can do.

Coffee ... just because

I put a pot of coffee on
just because I love you.
So you can sip
when you awake.
Just because I love you.

> *"Favorite time of day"*
> *is what you say*
> *coffee in the morning*
> *means to you.*

So I put a pot of coffee on
just because I love you.

You're dead tired — up
so late last night.
Now my work calls
with the morning light
... no time for me
    to drink coffee
    or to have a bit of
    brunch with you.

But I put a pot of coffee on
just because I love you.

> *"Favorite time of day"*
> *is what you say*
> *coffee in the morning*
> *means to you.*

So now I'm gone ...
and the coffee's on.
Just because I love you.

"Night owls" ...

... can coexist with "early risers" quite nicely, thank you.

And with more than one 'C'-mate living hundreds of miles away, I've spent many early evening as well as late night hours (you guessed it) on the phone.

'9 to 5' ... p.m. to a.m., that is

During one 26-day period, long-distance telecom records revealed that one 'C'-mate and I connected for 7,208 minutes. That's right: seven <u>thousand</u>. Figures out to an average of more than 4-1/2 hours ... every single day.

Our longest single phone conversation logged 487 minutes, from about 9:00 p.m. until after 5 a.m.

"What on earth do you two talk about?" people gasped.

"Everything" ...
from childhood days to what each of us was doing right now. And things we did <u>while talking</u> on the phone ran the gamut: cooking, washing dishes, sorting and folding laundry, getting dressed (or undressed) ...

> _"I'm putting my head through my shirt." (pause)_
> _"I'm pulling on my shorts ... If you hear a 'thud,'_
> _it's me — falling on the floor ...!"_

We also paid bills, flipped through magazines, put photos into albums (while recalling times and places from whence they came). And often at night, we sipped Scotch or wine.

We sang to each other, too ... along with CDs of many songs special to us ... relevant to our feelings (even now).

'You make me happy'
she said.

<u>I replied,</u>

I suggest, My Love, that

Happiness lives within You

*… just waiting for someone
to stop by and say,*

'Come out and play.'

There were also "moments" ...

... defined by my 'C'-mate as being totally focused on what we were saying/hearing. No multitasking allowed.

Topics for "moments" also ranged widely, from delivering exciting news of our day, to explaining reasons behind an attitude or action, "singing along" with music blaring from either (or both) stereo systems, and ... quietly murmuring highly intimate thoughts, wishes and desires.

"Moments," in short, provided prime times to connect.

And night after night, saying "Good night" was a lengthy and loving ritual.

Although you hate to hang up when you're "hung up," for Us the telephone "click" presaged special moments, too.

In the wee small hours ...

I slumbered in smiles

immersed
   in the echo
of your
gentle "good night" ...

... so far from you
... so close to you
     ... *with you*
cradled in my mind.

And maybe
(dare I wish it?)
   I was
cradled in yours.

Sleep well, my Love.
I'll be with you
when you wake.

Wherever you are.

<RES>

How you handle surprises

… can be a key to helping your relationship bloom fully and beautifully. Or it could, instead, throw a "hiccup" into the mix. (See "2nd-Thinking" – Chapter 5.)

And trust me, surprises there will be. Some, funny; some, disconcerting; some, just plain weird.

Some surprises may surprise both of you at once!

Like the time my 'C'-mate handed me the day's first mugful of coffee. Sweetened with "Chai Spice" or some other creamer that I'd had before (and liked), she anticipated (at the very least) "thank you" and a smile.

The thing is, I'm usually a black-coffee drinker — especially when starting my day. To make matters worse, when that mug arrived I was focused on paperwork of some sort.

I was not a "good sport."

My "what on earth is this? I drink coffee black" reaction surprised her, big-time. Not in a pleasant way.

Although we got over that "speed bump" (more or less), it raised a "red flag"… the kind of thing that could drive any 'C'-mate away.

The lesson here for Couples (I think) also applies to Life:

Be flexible. Be cool. Practice moderation — temper your responses to whatever happens, when.

Sometimes, however, when surprises rock your Couples boat, somewhat silly little things can ease tensions and brighten up your day …

Ever
'smoked a Twinkie®'?

We did. Twice.

30 seconds in a microwave:

watch what happens.

(Warning:

Let it cool before you eat

that sticky-sweet.)

"Good-morning" wake-up calls ...

can sometimes become an everyday thing. Even when (or, perhaps, especially when) you and your 'C'-mate are miles and miles apart.

I have awakened my sons, various coworkers and more than a few 'C'-mates over the years. In locations ranging from Denver, St. Augustine and Phoenix, to Cincinnati, Hartford (Connecticut), Washington, D.C., London and Madrid. Rockford and Grand Rapids, Michigan, too.

Not all Wake-up Calls by me are long-distance (praise be!). Oftentimes, the "Wake-_upee_" was slumbering in a nearby city or my own town; maybe just down the street.

Many, many times, I also functioned as a "snooze alarm" ... calling back again in 5-10 minutes or so, in order to help ease their way up-and-into the day.

And, since most people have their phones set to send callers to Voice Mail or an answering machine after "x" number of rings ... there were also mornings when my Wake-up _"Call"_ was more than just one.

caller #9

"Good morning."

At last — your voice
for real o'er the phone

   rather than
the recorded "Hi,
      this is …;
  leave a message
and I'll call you back."

After eight (count 'em — 8)
     voice mail messages,
  the 9th caller wins,
and
your "good morning" reminds me
what a fun time we had last night.
(Didn't we?)

Who knows when again?
Not we. Not yet.
  We'll
simply make times as we can.

One time
at a time.

© RES²

54

The best times for ...

getting to know each other, of course, are times when you actually are together.

Not just household-chore times or going-out times. But often (even better), spontaneous take-a-break or mini-getaway times.

One sunny Summer Saturday afternoon, for example, I mentioned to my 'C'-mate that a night club singer we had seen perform many years ago (she and I were with different partners then) ... was giving a one-time concert that evening at a riverside park 60 or so miles away.

We decided to drop our weekend errands and take a "scenic" 2-lane highway (vs. Interstate) drive ... enjoying the small-town countryside, while chatting non-stop about what we saw, as well as anything and everything else that popped into our heads.

The evening sunset concert amazed and enthralled us both. And an incredible full moon further mesmerized our eyes during the late-night, 2-lane highway drive home.

Whether or not you have memories such as this, invite your 'C'-mate to join you — and _make all-new ones_ ... times that create uniquely special memories for you.

They could come from something as simple as a walk in the park. A walk that could continue, in some ways, long after dark ...

"Good night" ... good day

"Just thought I'd say
          'Good night.'
...It was a really nice day
and I'm glad we talked..."

Yes, it was. Very nice.
All of it.

Our walk. Our talk.

Your voice right now.
Your call at 3 a.m.
and in-between...

Snuggling close and warm,
     cocooned in flannel
Your "first thing" morning
     client phone check
Soft caresses, unbridled passion
and the quiet comfort of our
     shared embrace

Mums along your driveway
Your house inside...now
     neatly dressed for home

Hiking shady trails
    on this sun-drenched Sunday
    afternoon

Picnic table by the mini-lake
An "ink stop"
    then
burgers 'n pie

Conversation, inspiration; Sharing
thoughts and
    hopes and fears...

    Relating.

Will your future,
            someday,
embrace "We"?
Intimately?
Fearlessly?

Answers in due time.
    For now...

...your call
brings a warm
        "Good night."

Hope it feels as good
for you to say it
as it does for me to hear it.

Once again ...

... a Communication Connection is crucial to any Couple relationship.

Hopefully, you have found that link by now. And it's time to move forward as a duo.

It can work just fine for you, even if some "traditional thoughts" don't as yet ring true.

I guess I Love You
(whatever that means)

It seems you want to hear
        three words
that don't come easy to me.

It's not because I don't care
    — that should be
plain to see.

It's just that I have seen
        those words
used so differently.

And I don't know how
    they can convey
all the things you are to me.

But I guess
I Love You
(whatever that means)

I guess
I Love You
(whatever that means)

Some men use
    three little words,
then disappear, next day.

Women, too,
    say "I love you,"
but just to get their way.

That's not for me.
        Can't you see
why those three words won't do?

I'm not like the rest!
        Yet I must confess
I don't know what else to do.

So I guess
I Love You
(whatever that means)

... *Yes, I guess*

I Love You

(whatever that means)

(A Missile in the Mail)

"I've got this little thing
I'd like to
share with you …"

"It's called
The Rest of My Life."

Chapter 3

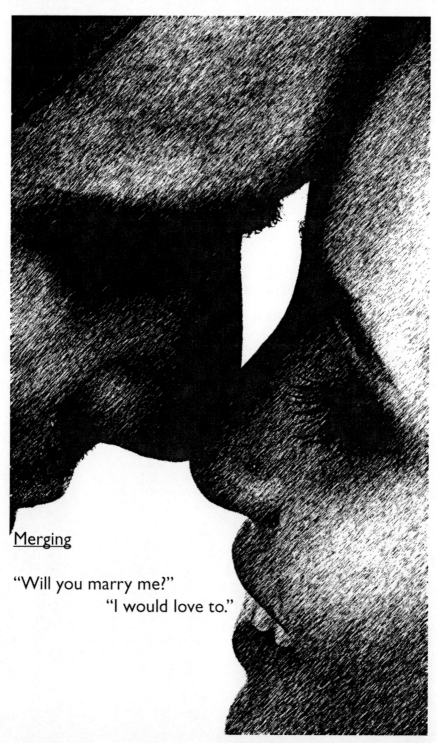

Merging

"Will you marry me?"
            "I would love to."

Although many Couples merge

… by simply living together, marriage is the ultimate step — and incorporates an element of commitment beyond other options.

Marriage (or the prospect thereof) also opens the way to exciting plans and activities — the wedding itself (date, venue, guests, bridesmaids and groomsmen, flowers, music …), plus prenuptial celebrations, honeymoon options — the works.

All of which offer opportunities for a Couple to share ideas as well as duties, strengthening their union-to-be.

All of which also can generate considerable stress.

Fact is, whether or not marriage is in the cards, moving in together — sharing a household — is almost certain to evoke a range of emotions back and forth, on a daily basis.

It's exciting and frightening — both at once.

Don't fight it; relish it!

Rejoice in the blend of anticipation, apprehension ... and let your Love know that you're bursting with feelings for him or her — and the joint journey you're taking ...

Let it remain

I'm tired
  Inspired
Excited
  Frighted
Happy
  Crappy
Hopeful
  Mopeful
Anxious
  Content
Confident
  Worry-bent
Casual
  Tensionful

Shooting high
  Plunging by
Dying slow. Living fast.
  On-the-go. Skidding past.
Penned. Loosed
  Asunder. Fused

Feel alive.
　　Have no drive
Unaware.
　　Strongly care
Flesh, bone here
　　Heart, soul there

Alone … no more
　　Heart sings. Heart-sore
Longing. Flirting
　　Laughing. Hurting
My life aglow
　　Midnight won't go

Empty. Filled
　　Born. Killed
Tearful. Elated
　　Sobered. Intoxicated

In Love?　　Insane?

Let it remain …

Treating each other ...

... with quiet, calm, measured understanding goes far toward alleviating fears inherent in virtually any Couple's merging of their households ... and their lives.

Being open, forthright & honest is crucial. (Remember that word "trust" noted in "Finding your 'C'-mate"?)

This starts, of course, long before you reach the stage you're at now. But "back then," many personal details, physical features or foibles didn't seem to be important. After all, you were only "dating."

(Note: We're not talking past girlfriends & boyfriends here; although we'll touch on that, too.)

You may have a surgical scar, for example (I do), or dental issues or a tattoo (what? where?) — things your 'C'-mate hasn't noticed, or at least hasn't indicated he/she has.

Suddenly, stark reality rears it's ugly head in the form of potential embarrassment ... fear of "exposure."

Don't panic. What's the worst that can happen when he or she finds out? They tell you "Good-by"? (OK — bad example; that's not what you want.)

First of all, don't be surprised to learn that they already know — but don't mind at all, or didn't want to comment for fear of embarrassing you!

Or they may say, when you tell them, "Really? Can I see?" ... which, in the right situation, could be fun.

How do you bring up the subject? How do you find out?

It isn't every day

… that you find yourself
in a carpeted Master bathroom,
wearing only your jockey shorts
and your 'C'-mate says

'Lay down.
I want to look
inside
your mouth.'

But, hey — she was
a dental hygienist, so I figured
it would be OK.

In fact, by the time she finished, it was kinda fun!

Chances are, you and your 'C'-mate will opt for other
places and methods to broach sensitive issues.
For example …

Making a 'game'...

... out of discussing potentially embarrassing topics can ease-open the door.

It could take the form of a "True Confessions" night over a glass of wine (heck — make it a bottle, and have a backup handy). Or "let's play 'Worst Case Scenario': what's the worst thing you think I might learn about you, when we're living together?" ... "And vice versa." ... "I'll go first."

You may begin with something less than the "worst." And take turns, of course.

> _Listening_
> _is the first half of_
> _speaking._
>
> _Actually, it may be_
> _90 percent._

Once you get into these subjects, tensions ease quickly and you'll have a great time not only exchanging information, but also learning ideals and attitudes that could bring you closer.

The same thing applies when discussing 'most anything. Including your past "love lives." The mere fact that the two of you are "discussing" may be a major plus vs. past partners ...

'It's so absolutely

wonderful

to be talked to

and cared for and

listened to …'

Former girlfriends/boyfriends ...

... or former spouses are typically "the big issue" with merging Couples — although this often is dealt with at an earlier relationship stage.

Sometimes, parental issues from childhood leave emotional or attitudinal scars still today.

To be sure, if you've known each other for a long time, have a "family history" or similar links, you already know (and presumably accept) various issues that could present unwelcome surprises among Couples who have more recently met.

On the other hand, to me it's not necessary to know everything about your partner's past. After all, it is "history." Your view of each other and where you're headed as a Couple now is far more important.

But it never hurts to ask — especially if you really want to know. Hopefully, you can handle whatever you find out.

Here again, openness and honesty are key. And that cuts both ways, for both of you.

As you learn, chances are new issues will emerge. But by now you can better communicate — and resolve them.

With all this "togetherness" going on, remember ...

Alone-times are important, too.

And sometimes, simple gestures like a late night phone call after an evening of "discussing things" can generate very good feelings, both ways ...

I arrived home ...

My telephone message machine said:

"Monday, 12-oh-1 a.m."

And her voice said:
"Hi, it's me. Naturally, I'm wide awake now ..."
(A few words about our evening), then:

"... You have to do a lyric for moonlight
('cause) it's like daylight in my bedroom.
Have a good sleep; talk to you tomorrow."

Monday, at 6:40 a.m., I gave her this ...

lovesent

It's one minute after midnight.
"Like daylight" in your room.
A quiet chill
      creeps o'er the hill
and my arms left too soon
         to carry you to slumber
with a gentle, warm embrace.
   I lift my eyes
   up to the skies
and send you in my place ...

   "Moonday" ... what a way
         to ease into the week.
   Please weave sweet dreams
         with soft-white beams
   and cradle her to sleep.

My call will come too early
   (as it does any morn);
tomorrow you must hurry
   to conquer worlds anon.
I wish that I could be there
to hold you, help you rest.
   For now, I send
   a special friend
with wishes heaven-blessed ...

   "Moonday" ... what a way
         to ease into the week.
   Please weave sweet dreams
         with soft-white beams
   and cradle her to sleep.

   "Moonday" ... what a way
         to ease into the week.
   Please weave sweet dreams
         with soft-white beams
   and cradle her ...

Sometimes divorce

… opens the way for a Couple to truly share a life, whether or not they marry. It can also offer opportunity for gestures such as …

The "Freedom Bouquet,"
 a congratulatory flower arrangement sent one time, the day after she told me a settlement had been reached.

>*"Welcome to the Springtime of Your New Life,"*
>my note read. *"Here's hoping that it grows brighter,*
>*more beautiful and enjoyable with each and every*
>*season, every single day."*

It was well received. And, not so incidentally, the wishes that I expressed, continue to come true.

Of course, getting involved with recent divorcees can raise eyebrows along with comments about "on the rebound," "it's too soon," "he (or she) needs more time" and so forth.

And if, perchance, things don't work out between you, the I-told-you-so crowd is quick to speak. <u>My reply</u>:

> *"Revel in the Wonder*
> *of newfound Love*
> *... and the*
> *Memories in its Wake."*

I've experienced this firsthand; one situation, in particular.

I submit, for openers, that nay-sayers' over-generalizing fails to recognize the depth of true Couple feelings — whether or not their relationship becomes permanent.

As I noted earlier: "If it feels right to you, it's the right thing to do." I still feel that way.

'I have lived and
been treated like
a princess
during my marriage.

But I
never felt like one
until you came along.'

When you truly care ...

... it shows. In the words you use, the tone of your voice, the moves you make — in short, the way you treat each other, day after day after day.

It goes without saying (but I will, anyway) that it matters not a bit if your 'C'-mate has been single all of his or her life, is a product of divorce or other, less-formal prior relationships.

To be sure, your particular background, past experiences and lifestyle lead to habits and mannerisms, or provide perspectives that may differ from those of your 'C'-mate.

As a result, one of you could be taken aback, feel hurt or embarrassed by the other's comments or actions in a professional business setting, a social or family gathering — or even when it's just the two of you.

No need to panic. Roll with it as smoothly as you can (if "in public") and address it later, in private. Recount the occurrence clearly and calmly, explain what you found bothersome, and why. If there's a corrective "fix" you can suggest, by all means do so.

If the issue is more complex, discussion can lead you to one or more agreeable ways to do things "next time."

Whether resolving issues or simply enjoying life, you will (hopefully) feel an ever-stronger connection ... including more-intimate times.

These could be considered a sequel to "love at first sight," e.g. "Love at first touch." Times like these may also reveal 'C'-mate nuances — lovely, endearing nuances, at that ...

loveblush

Please
don't ask the red to go
— Nature's
rich rose rouge
         resplendent
   in your cheeks
  from the love
we just made …

Ever been to ...

... a garden wedding? I almost starred in one. (But that's another story.)

Idyllic, such ceremonies can be. Sunshine. Blue sky. Maybe a harp and a flute greeting guests and accompanying vows. With shade trees and flowers — acres of them, everywhere.

On the other hand, one of the loveliest ceremonies I've attended, took place in a small courtroom. It was a warm Autumn day on a Friday the 13th — perhaps, the most colorful Autumn-leaf October I can remember.

But nothing tops the intimacy of another Friday the 13th ceremony (yes, I like to defy superstition) ... marking my one and only marriage to-date. It took place in our apartment, with a few close friends and family. We exchanged personally written vows, which didn't include "I do."

The union lasted 20 years. (But that's another story, too.)

Point is: Whatever the venue and however you plight your troth — whether simple or elaborate, a short ceremony or long — it's yours and yours alone.

And that makes it very special, indeed.

"The only thing
I see exceeding
how I feel about you today
is how I will feel
about you tomorrow.

And the next day.

And the next,
and ..."

The Wedding CD

Music typically plays a role as Couples get to know one another and form more permanent alliances. Especially when their alliance reads "w-e-d-d-i-n-g."

There's the "Signature Song" to which the bride and groom dance at their wedding reception. It may be a song that was playing when they first met or became engaged, or which in some other way is especially significant to them.

Some Couples put several songs relating to their relationship on a CD, and give them as "favors" to wedding guests.

I know of one Couple for whom music went far beyond this — virtually defining much of what went on in their lives as their relationship evolved. They selected 20-some songs ... "messages of love, caring and commitment" ... to be compiled in a Wedding CD unrivaled anywhere.

I don't recall hearing that their CD actually came to be.

I guess I wasn't invited to the wedding.

flow'r garden melodies

It seemed just like a fairy tale,

    the joining of we two

    in an ultra-scenic setting.

Friends 'n family thought so, too.

Superbly manicured gardens

    filled with flowers 'n trees;

sunshine, blue sky and

music wafting in the breeze …

Now that garden setting,

with you 'n me

becoming We

    — just like a fairy tale,

transcends reality.

'Happy New Home,'

the card read. "May it be a place filled with sunshine and smiles." I added the thought "forever and for always," with a fuzzy, stuffed two-puppy toy that said "Kiss me" when squeezed.

We sipped the previous home owner's gift of *Dom Perignon* on move-in day. Vintage 1988.

Regardless, the message here is quite simple:

Whether it's hers or his or, ideally, "ours" — do a little something to make that new house or apartment a *cause celebre*. A 6-pack, cheese 'n crackers will do.

If nothing else, it gives you a welcome break from supervising the movement of furnishings, clothes and boxes (tons of boxes) — or carrying it all yourself.

After a long day of moving, in most households (actually, I suspect, in virtually <u>all</u>) the first piece of furniture to be fully assembled is ... the bed.

Although the rigors of the day make a good night's sleep priority #1, the <u>excitement</u> of those rigors finally and fully bringing you two together could, perhaps, delay your "good night's sleep" a bit.

duet

Come to me. I'm your
     Maiden Fair.
Lovingly, I'll teach you to care.
   I will make you a man
   like you've never been.

With my lips,
my fingertips
and gentle as a dove
   ... untamed,
     unashamed
I'll give you love.

     Where did you learn to love,
       Maiden Fair?
     When will you once more
     take me there?
     You make me a man
     like I've never been.
     With your lips,
     your fingertips
     and gentle as a dove
       ... untamed,
         unashamed
     you give me love.

Come to me. I'm your
     Maiden Fair.
Lovingly, I'll teach you to care.

     You make me a man
     like I've never been.

With my lips,
my fingertips
and gentle as a dove
   ... untamed,
     unashamed
I give you love.

© RES[2]

The Boudoir.

Whether married or not, a Couple's overnight environment can go far toward enhancing togetherness. And it can be as varied as Couples themselves.

Candles bring warm color and soft, sensual light to virtually any bedroom, regardless of furnishing style or size.

Candles also add extraordinary ambience around Master Bath tubs — strategically placed, of course, to prevent dousing when Couples relax amid piles of bubbles after, say, pulling weeds from flowerbeds on a hot Summer day.

My candle enviro-experiences range from single to multiple candle colors, shapes, scents, sizes & styles — from tiny tea-light candles to towering candelabra and/or huge self-standing masses of wax with wicks.

Speaking of wax ... here's a candle tip: Burning candles drip, leaving globs of hardened wax that can be tough to scrape up. I'm told that the culprit is paraffin; and that *paraffin-free* candles leave drippings that clean up with ease — making for a more pleasant "morning after."

Meanwhile in the Boudoir ... comforters, sheets, pillow cases, shams — all carry patterns and colors and textures that project 'most any visual impression a Couple desires.

I've had the good fortune to enjoy rather warm, subdued ambiences (the intimacy of which I normally prefer) as well as some far bolder or even a bit risqué.

Fact is, Love ...   *Any Boudoir will do*
                when it's for me and you.

The bed itself.

My past has included nothing more than a relatively slim mattress on an apartment floor. But hey — when it's the two of you ... who's complaining?

I spent many a loving night in a single bed, too. Cozy as can be, especially on cold Midwestern winter nights.

My own double bed has staunchly weathered too many years. I love the bookcase headboard for stashing a pad, pen, flashlight, box of tissues 'n stuff — while sometimes catching "flack" for an aging, too-thin mattress that occasionally creaks "to the rhythm of the night ..."

Queen seems to be the standard size nowadays for most folks.

And thanks to one 'C'-mate once upon a time, I know what it means to "climb into bed."

Hers was huge. King-plus, I guess. Plenty of room to roam side-to-side. More to the point: the deep-deep thick mattress could closely match the entire stack of mattresses in "The Princess and the Pea."

First time there, I looked for a safety net.

Fortunately, we spent most of our waking moments as well as sleep time sharing (you guessed it) the middle.

In any case, I hope that the bed that works best for me, also works best for you, to wit:

Whichever bed you share with the One you Love.

With a few fluid moves, she pulled off
her top ... stepped out of her jeans ...
and threw a quizzical glance my way.

'So ... ?'

Seconds later, I softly replied.

'You wear the sexiest

undergarments in the world.

You are the most sensuous

woman alive.

The combination is breathtaking.'

She smiled.

Pillow talk

Pillows are quite the thing in some Boudoirs. I remember one that had more pillows than any sleepyhead needs.

She had "Show Pillows": thick Euro-style cushions and shams. Three of 'em; each a good 24" - 30" square. They were removed each night before climbing into bed; replaced along the headboard each morning when the bed was made. A classy, striking look — I must say.

She had "Petite Pillows," about as wide as my forearm is long. The "babies" among the bed's pillow family, they were just-for-show, too.

And, yes, we also had "Sleep Pillows" — over-sized, standard-shape cushions of comfort upon which to rest our heads.

All coverings matched and/or complemented, of course. Beautifully. When the bed was made and it all came together, its invitation was clear:

"Jump in and enjoy ..."

Snuggled in the middle, between the two "Sleep" pillows was a mid-size "maverick." Softer and scrunchier than any of the others, my Love claimed this pillow as hers — totally. She laughingly guarded it with unabashed intensity ... said it marked her Territory, and woe to me if I trespassed.

She also had no qualms "crossing the border":
With that pillow, we spent the majority (by far) of our most passionately intimate, memorable love-making moments.

In oh-so many ways, it was for Us, **The Love Pillow**.

"Nothing could make me happier than to have your child.

"That would be the greatest gift I could give you."

The mere thought

… of having a baby can chill many Couple's ardor; understandably so.

Far sadder are situations where a Couple wants to conceive, but for one reason or another is unable to do so. This can create even more anxiety, stress and unhappiness than an unwanted pregnancy.

Fortunately for most Couples — at least among those inclined to have a family — the expressed desire to "have your child" enhances actual, *physical* desire.

Now the thought of creating a new life together, stirs deeper emotions and more intense sensuality than any other idea imaginable.

This is also true, in my experience, among Couples who discover each other when childbearing and rearing are behind them. Whether it's pleasant memories from their individual pasts, or the depth of their feelings for each other now (actually, I suspect it's both) …

… the thought of how wonderful it could be to conceive as a Couple, lifts their physical as well as emotional togetherness even higher.

It's a level of caring and sharing unequalled anywhere.

caremaking

Excited ... entranced ... enraptured
by your touch
          my heart races,
          my head feels light
in ways I haven't felt since
... since ... youth (?)
"A kid," if you will.
              No!
Not so.
I'm not a kid.
Nor do I wish to be.

A kid
(at least the kid I once was
and others I've known)
couldn't
care for you
          as I do
couldn't feel for you
          as I do
couldn't touch you
          as I do
with passion
that
lingers ... savors ...
soothes as it excites
relaxes and awakens
          all at once

unhurried
un-harried.

A kid
would "enter"
rather than wait
          for you
to draw me in ...
and
would miss
the ultimate ecstasy
   of Invitation
in lieu of conquest.

A kid
couldn't
become gentler, slower
quieter, more at ease
    — even as hearts
pound faster,
breath grows shorter
and satin-smooth skin
tingles for more ...

A kid
couldn't pause
to hold you,
simply hold you

or to listen
... hear you
       murmur
"touch me more
    ... it feels so good"
   and truly share
your desire

"caremaking"
the pleasure of making love
*   to the nth degree.*

It tells you
someone wants
       you
really wants you
   all of you
as you are ...

A kid,
you see,
wants pleasure
       but doesn't yet
understand that

pleasure is a gift.
And a gift
must first be given.

Chapter 4

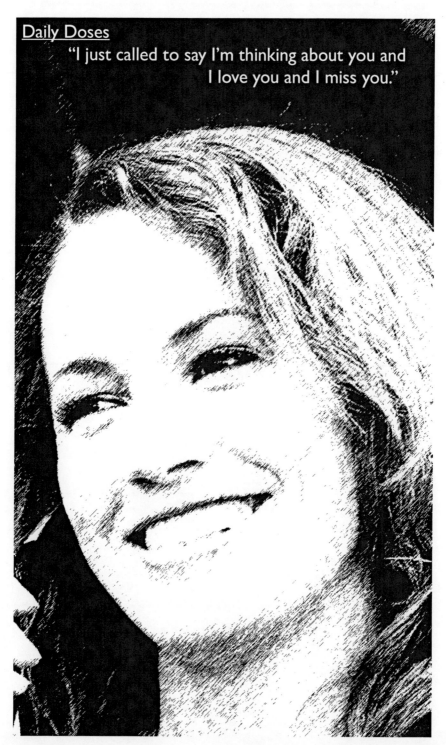

Daily Doses

"I just called to say I'm thinking about you and
I love you and I miss you."

Wouldn't it be great ...

to get home (or turn on your cell phone) and hear your 'C'-mate's smiling voice?

Trust me: It is.

Mini echoes resonate maxi impact — not only as a first-time surprise, but also again and again. Maybe with a subtle twist, at a different time ... whatever.

Even if your day's not going well (or especially when it's not), it helps to pick up the phone or turn to your 'C'-mate and say something nice. "Hi" all by itself is a fine place to start.

It's the kind of thing that makes someone smile. What's more, it takes far fewer muscles to smile than to frown.

And smiles make any day brighter for all.

The Smile Song

There just ain't no easy way
to get by in life today,
    except with a smile
    and a song.

Every time I turn around
everybody wears a frown
    'til they start
    to sing along:

    Ain't life grand
when you've got a friend or two
…whether rich or poor,
    old or new.
Though I can't afford my rent,
bein' friends don't cost a cent.
    I'm so glad
    to be with you!

Workin' drives me up a wall.
Money don't go far at all.
    My wealth is a smile
    and a song.

Though I'm careful what I spend,
who knows where it all will end?
    I'll just smile…
    and sing along!

    Ain't life grand
when you've got a friend or two
…whether rich or poor,
    old or new.
Though I can't afford my rent,
bein' friends don't cost a cent.
    I'm so glad
    to be with you!

(Repeat Chorus)

© RES & THS[5]

There's much to do ...

... in any household — even an apartment, condo or townhouse with no yard work involved.

And to-do's offer opportunity for Couples to share as well as "divvy up" duties, making chores go quickly and more pleasantly.

Although the instinct is to have one or the other of you do those chores following traditional male/female roles, or based on what he/she "is good at" — make an effort to flip those coins, at least now and then. You can teach each other something new, or how to do it better, faster.

One 'C'-mate taught me quicker, easier ways to clean the bathtub and shower. A formerly dreaded task now gets done more frequently. And, yes, better.

Laundry tips. Cooking techniques. Bed-making methods (that's right).

It's fun to teach and to learn. And genuine feelings of accomplishment flow both ways.

That also goes for outdoor stuff,

… if your home's in such a venue.

Vegetable gardening brings some Couples multiple rewards, from planting through harvest.

Birds or other neighborhood wildlife offer potential, with special houses and feed — also selected flowers to create, for example, a sanctuary for Hummingbirds.

Even pulling weeds can be enlightening and (somewhat) fulfilling. One weekend, a 'C'-mate turned me on to simple tools 'n techniques …

> _"You've got to get_
> _the roots out."_

Then she got P-O'ed as I finished digging out a patch of thistles after sunset — when she was ready to quit. Go figure.

Her point wasn't lost, however.

Although time spent doing chores can be rewarding, there comes the time for "calling it a day."

And there are ways to make those times especially meaningful, too.

Togetherness Times...

...go fine with wine
　　　Italian style
and other sips that help
　　　you smile

Times to sit and talk,
(or stand or walk)
to laugh and think and
nurture dreams

　— away
from work and
daily stress,
times like these
can ease duress;

　shut out
the haze of hectic days
　(but still within
　the life you lead)

Oases…
where you each can heed
thoughts that told you
    "yes, I care"
along with fresh ideas to share;
to carry you from here
    to there

Together…ness Times.

Even when life's clock
    may seem to say
"it's too late"
    I hope you find
        (better still)
"create"

Togetherness Times
    to uncover smiles,
    to clear your view

    Discover evermore
your own unique
"me, we and you."

Birthdays, Holidays ...

... anniversaries, of course (wedding, when you met, became engaged) ... many special occasions offer mutual moments in which Couples can enhance their relationships — while also easing the stress that often _accompanies_ such occasions.

Addressing Christmas cards or party invitations together — or "save-the-date" and wedding invitations — can be a great way to spend an evening or three. A little wine can help make these times special occasions, too.

Brainstorming gifts for family and friends can be a hoot. And, closer to home ... staying tuned to each other's likes provides a steady stream of ideas: Tickets to sporting events, concerts and theatre, CDs & DVDs; spa treatments and other more personal items, too.

If, for instance, one (or both) of you enjoy dancers on TV ("Gee, wish I could move like that!") ... dance lessons could be the perfect gift. And 'twould be "a gift that keeps on giving," as you enjoy times together on the dance floor more and more.

'Foreplay' for the day

"There is nothing finer

than waking up

with you beside me,

holding you close

and whispering ...

'Good morning, Luv.' "

While anniversaries and such

… are occasions that you share, the anniversary of your 'C'-mate's birth gives you a special day to say "I care."

Several especially exciting birthdays come to my mind. Two in particular, stand out:

The first involves a 'C'-mate's Day.

Gifts, for the most part, followed traditional lines: A Swarovski collectible relating to a childhood hobby of hers. Dinner, and theatre tickets to a musical she'd been wanting to see.

But the biggest hit (some may not agree) was when I entered the bedroom on her Birthday morn, carrying a Red Velvet layer cake emblazoned with "Happy New Year" … and a handwritten sign that read:

"Life
is short.
Eat dessert first."

Birthday cake for breakfast never tasted so good.

The second standout was for my Day.
She gave me an extraordinary watch, as well as several books, personal items & more — and a weekend seashore getaway to a place I'd never been before. We logged many uniquely special togetherness times during those several days.

Ultimately, she left — and took my heart.

I kept the Rolex.

106

It's tough to top

... a warm smile, an embrace and a cheery "Hi, Luv" when stepping into your home or apartment.

The sound of music, however, livens up any arrival — and the rest of your evening, too. Rock, country, classical, blues — whatever you choose can set or enhance the mood. And, as the saying goes, "variety is the spice ...": don't hesitate to vary the sounds you enjoy.

Of course, there's much more than music. Paintings, sculptures, photos as well as colors, shapes and patterns on walls, furnishings and elsewhere — all stimulate the senses and help keep daily life alive, fresh, interesting.

And you don't have to be an art aficionado or a singer or a musician to admire and enjoy — or to add a karaoke-style performance to your surroundings *d' jour.*

Some people turn environmental stimulation into creative artistry — a phenomenon in the case of one Couple, which led me to the term "Inspiration Situation."

You know what? *They're just having a good time*!

So can you. I've seen firsthand how simple give-and-take sparks a dynamic that strengthens their Couple-ship in very real ways. Check it out: an inspiration to us all ...

Me 'n you

Is it the man and his music
— the melody? ...
awakening
        the imagery
I put into words so vividly?
    It really matters not
    because, you see,

It's Inspiration
    Situation.

Is it her laugh? Her eyes? Her grace?
Her wit? ... urging my fingers onto keys,
creating multiple melodies?
    Whatever it is,
    I go with it.

It's Inspiration
    Situation.

Rhymes and music, musings and tunes
sometimes grow in harmony — sometimes
they flow separately, lifting us
to heights anew ...

    Created by me.
    Inspired by you.

It seems the more we share our daily
fare ... trials that could drive us away,
blend with triumphs and bid us "stay."
The place for me and you
is with we two

    ... Inspiration
        Situation.

Recipe for Spice

Creativity can take many forms throughout your home. For example: Pick a routine entrée — any entrée: beef, perhaps; a type of seafood or, one from my life: chicken breasts.

"Here's a newspaper feature with a dozen ways to liven up chicken breasts: sautéed with cherry-shiraz sauce ... skillet-poached with tarragon-lemon beurre blanc ... pan-fried with mushroom-chardonnay ... panko crusted with cilantro vinaigrette ... Creole three-pepper garden chicken ...

"If we try one of these just once a month, we could enjoy a 'new' chicken entrée for an entire year."

I was excited. My 'C'-mate seemed willing, but it hasn't yet come to pass.

Regardless, you get the idea. And maybe it'll work for you.

In the process, you can spice up your "Life around the island."

Life around the island

It may not be an island in the sun.
In our home it was an island of fun.
No sandy beach or seaside view;
just a "getaway" spot for me 'n you.

Sipping cocktails. Prepping brunch,

hors d'oeuvres for a party ...

Or today's special: Dinner for two.

And breakfasts: love-in-the-morning culinary marvels.

It's the hub of life in many kitchens: the island with a stovetop

on one side, a counter and (maybe) bar stools on the other —

perfect setting for an evening, morning or anytime getaway from

the hubbub of elsewhere life.

What a place to enjoy together!

Your home kitchen has no "island"? No problem. Consider the wall-side countertop your seashore — just the place for doing all of the same things, and more.

Of course, my 'C'-mates typically were (by far) the better chefs. My last fiancée was a whiz with complex recipes, multiple seasonings 'n stuff. With her, there was no such thing as "plain."

Yet, once in a while I score a *coup*. Like with Pork Chops in Wine Sauce, a simple rich-tasting dish, the recipe for which came from my Mother. I also know that the best way to "cut through" egg whites to remove a piece of shell or whatever … is with the egg shell itself!

But with 'C'-mates, cooking isn't a contest. At least it never has been with us. Don't let it be with you.

Two for Two

For Couples, dinner and breakfast/brunch pretty much dominate in-home dining. Here's a simple recipe for each. These options also come with major plusses for amateurs like me:

- Few ingredients
- Few dishes to wash
- Minimal "active" prep time

Richly Romantic Dinner: Pork Chops in Wine Sauce**

Ingredients:
- Pork Chops (4; boneless, butterfly cut)
- Cream of Mushroom soup (three 10-1/2 oz cans)
- Tawny Port wine (approx. two cups*)

Steps: (Total prep time = 15-20 minutes)
1. Brown pork chops in skillet with butter; season with
   salt & pepper
   While browning chops …
2. * Mix soup with wine (just a bowl & whisk; *"eye-ball" wine amount … 'til sauce is richly Tawny, not too runny)
3. Place browned chops in butter-greased pan
4. Pour wine sauce over chops, cover with foil and bake at 350° F for about 90 minutes

Enjoy each other's company while you wait.

** Goes great with baked potato (sauce makes tasty "gravy")

After an enjoyable evening … ease into the morning:

Go with an upscale option that I _love_ and often order when brunching in a restaurant — because I never make it at home. Perhaps I will, starting now.

Morning-after Brunch: Eggs Benedict*

Ingredients:
- English muffins (two, split into flat halves)
- Canadian Bacon (aka ham) (4 slices)
- Eggs (4; we prefer Jumbo)
- Hollandaise Sauce

"The secret is in the sauce," a gourmet Chef tells me. "Careful with the lemon; most people overdo it." He suggests that amateurs like me avoid from-scratch in favor of package-based. "Best from the pack is Knorr — it's fool-proof," says he. Says me, "Done."

Steps: (Prep time = 15-20 minutes; plus 5 min. cook time)
1. **Poach eggs** (3-4 min. for soft center, runny yolk; 5-7 min. for slightly cooked center, firm white)
2. Cook/Fry Can. bacon/ham (slowly; not too brown or dry)
3. Toast English muffins
4. Prep Hollandaise
   - Whisk sauce mix & 1 cup milk in saucepan
   - Add 1/4-cup margarine or butter & bring to a boil, stirring frequently
   - Reduce heat and simmer, stirring until thick (~ 1 min.)

5. Serve-up the combo: muffin half + "bacon" +
      poached egg ... topped by your Hollandaise

A mighty tasty way to begin a Sunday. Or any other day.

    *   Tomato Juice makes a superb Benedict companion.
      Especially if you add a tad of Worcestershire, a dash
      of Tabasco, and sprinkle a bit of pepper on top.
You can also "vodka-ize" it into a Bloody Mary ... garnished with
a stick of celery or (my favorite) a kosher dill pickle slice.

What about you …

… in the kitchen? Gourmet chef? Or one whose dinner skills start/stop with "making reservations"?

Chances are, from somewhere or time, you have a Signature Recipe of some sort.

By all means, prepare it for (or with) your 'C'-mate. To mark a special occasion, or to make any occasion special. Just for the two of you.

How about finding your own "Couple" Signature Recipe — a new, special entrée you've never had before?

Trying different, interesting options in search of The One could, in itself, provide many good times along the way.

Of course, before you do the cooking, you have to do the shopping. And that can be a mighty-fun thing, too.

The supermarket song

Just up the aisle from the Cheerios
— past the tea and coffee brown,
stands the store Deli
where special meats 'n cheese
'n salad stuff abound.

Next comes the pasta, sauces and
rows 'n rows of vegetables.
   A few steps more
    and it's a picnic store
— right down to fresh Kaiser rolls!

   Supermarket walkin';
   what a great way to be.
   The price of food may go sky-high
   — but I still can look for free!

I wear a smile down the dairy aisle
filled with butter, milk and cheese,
      yogurt, eggs 'n all;
    then I gaze in awe
at frozen foods displayed for me:

Fruit juice, ice cream, pizza pies,
waffles, spinach, broccoli …
         Next, a change of pace
         at the fresh meat case
with a host of cuts to see!

   Supermarket walkin';
   what a great way to be.
   The price of food may go sky-high
   — but I still can look for free!

I wouldn't miss a week of this.
Supermarkets are a trip!
         Always something new
         watching shoppers, too.
But long checkout lines I skip!

   Supermarket walkin';
   what a great way to be.
   The price of food may go sky-high
   — but I still can look for free!

One 'C'-mate of mine ...

... had a knack for turning a 5-minute store stop ("let's pick up some ground beef on sale") ... into a 50-minute quest involving side dishes, appetizers, seasonings 'n spices — the works.

This typically <u>also</u> led to an hour of so of meal making, rather than 15-minutes-and-done.

Has this happened to you? If so, you may (as I initially did) find it frustrating — especially after a long day when you simply want to get home, sit down and eat.

But I couldn't help but marvel as she pieced together dishes and ingredients on-the-fly, traversing store aisles with intensity and excitement that I never before knew.

And every dinner was a feast for the senses — eyes, ears, nose, taste buds and all.

With her, no meal was mundane. And I loved her for it. Matter of fact, I still do.

All of this vastly expanded my Supermarket acumen, too. Got so I could even locate the _Cilantro_ on my own.

In short, it's a learning process — about each other and tasks that are part of your life, every day.

So roll with it! Take the lead, or follow your partner's.

It'll make your Couple-times more fun, more satisfying ... more worthwhile.

Things to "look forward to"

A part of enjoying everyday life could be planning "big times" together.

Maybe your honeymoon, if you're not yet married. Or a vacation. Or a road trip with friends. Or …?

Stimulated, perhaps, by things on TV or articles you see or something someone else did — a myriad of options can be bandied about.

You'll find some, no doubt, that pique your interest, suit your schedule and budget.

Maybe short-term, quick jaunts to all-new or "old favorite" haunts: Three-day Vegas weekends, bed 'n breakfast overnights, as well as day-trip apple picking and Christmas tree cutting — options abound for any weekend, any season, any time.

Given a week or two or longer, plus enough bucks, lengthy cruises or overseas travel give you even more to think about and plan for.

Like a Safari vacation in Africa. I know folks who have done it; such a trip including me was also mentioned a time or two.

In the process of bringing plans like this to fruition, a local zoo or amusement park could provide a "sneak preview" …

Safari down the street ...

An African safari — what
a vacation that would be!
    New sights and sounds
    where animals abound
and other things
that we have yet to see.

The Giraffes, they say,
anytime (night or day)
    stick their heads
    right into your tent.
But — wait, you say ...

No time or money
to do it now, Honey?
No problem.
Here's something really neat.

    Before our big getaway,
    let's ride an Elephant today!
At the "Safari down the street."

She's a sweet elephant who
    would love to take me 'n you
for a brief stroll or more.
Then we could watch her paint art,
    play harmonica — so smart!
And feed her ice cream, hay 'n
vegetables galore.

It's within easy reach,
and a fun place to meet.
    Com' on — let's go see.
    Ride the elephant with me!
At the "Safari down the street."

Bored? Games ...

... can provide a pleasant diversion any evening, on a lazy Sunday or rainy afternoon. Even with just the two of you.

There are tons from which to choose: Monopoly, Scrabble and other standards. Checkers and chess (your chance to re-enact the intimate interplay between Faye Dunaway and Steve McQueen in the original "Thomas Crown Affair").

Card games, too: Uno, poker, black jack, rummy, bridge and more, including euchre (left, right or best "bower," anyone?)

New games as well as "updates" arrive *en masse* prior to every Christmas holiday — gift ideas that can add to fun-times, too.

Gaming at casinos can be enjoyed 'most anywhere or any time — no Vegas or Atlantic City trip needed.

game works

Roll the dice.
Deal the cards.
Make your move.
   Lots of games
put us in the groove.

Pick an eve,
a rainy day
— me and you
can break away
   to have a little fun.

Somehow,
the work will get done

And doing it
will be more fun, too!

© RES

Thoroughbred racing ...

... when a track's nearby is a fun way to spend a sunny afternoon.

Dog races can be a hoot, too. Bet on the rabbit — it
always wins.

There's drag racing, stock cars, demo derbies or Formula
One ... A Couple I know (and they're not alone) is into tractor
pulls, big time.

Given the time and money, you could take up golf. Or in your
yard or a nearby park, play horseshoes or croquet.

Here, there, everywhere — leisure options abound. All your
'C'-mate and you need to do is choose a few ... and go.

Enjoy the aftermath, too.

'Twas the table

by the window ...

at Las Palmas, shortly after the last
horserace was run.

Margaritas.
Chips & Salsa.
Enchiladas.

And you.
Occasionally peering o'er the top of
your glasses, intently calculating how
much you won. Or lost.

Acoustic guitar notes drew near.

And you talked about Madrid and
practiced your Spanish with the
strolling *mariachi* in-between
nostalgic, romantic serenades.

We vowed to spend a day this way
again.

... Just say "when."

Magnetic attraction

It started as a cluttered collection of decorative magnets sprawled across the refrigerator door.

She removed most. Rearranged a few.

Then she proceeded to disassemble a sizable magnet comprised of individual words and a few short terms.

At first I wondered. What now? More of a mess?

Then I marveled.

When I next entered the kitchen, a few mini messages adorned the white fridge door.

> "Be cool"   "I want you"
> A tiny love-heart
> "Great Together"

Wow. Simple, powerful, meaningful statements. Collectively conveying an even bigger message:

Unclutter your fridge door … your mind … your life.

'When you lean on me

you tell me

that I'm important.'

There's nothing quite like "being there" for each other.
And no one else is quite like the one who's there for you.

In bad times and sad times, mad times and glad times — any time.
And in so many unwritten ways.

While major crises leap to the fore (major illness or accident,
a family member's death; loss of job, terrorist attack, natural
disaster; spouse's infidelity, divorce …) "being there" for your
'C'-mate encompasses many relatively minor-but-meaningful
aspects of daily life.

Contact may be face-to-face, via phone or whatever.
The point is: Contact. Listening, perhaps questioning or
suggesting … communicating. Being there.

It was summed up rather nicely by one 'C'-mate of mine when,
near the end of our phone-talk she said:

> *"Thanks for letting me vent.*
> *You're good.*
> *For me. And with me."*

Hopefully, you and your 'C'-mate will feel this way, too.

for a little while ...

Y' know how sometimes
you just want to lose yourself in
someone's arms and
be held and
feel cared for ...
that someone is there
and the rest of the world
— for a little while,
at least — doesn't matter;
only you.

That's how I feel
so often
when you call
— even if it's to "complain" and
relieve your frustration over
something you heard
or that someone did
... or you feel
a bit swamped with
an overdose of daily life.

By time the call ends, you are
laughing and rejuvenated and
back on a roll.
Me, too.

It only gets better
when we are together,
caring and sharing for real.
    Either way,

It's one of the many things we do
for each other …

    like no one else
        ever has,
or ever can.

Which makes you and me and,
    yes, We
extraordinary.

To be treasured and nurtured
for a long,
    long … while.

Chapter 5

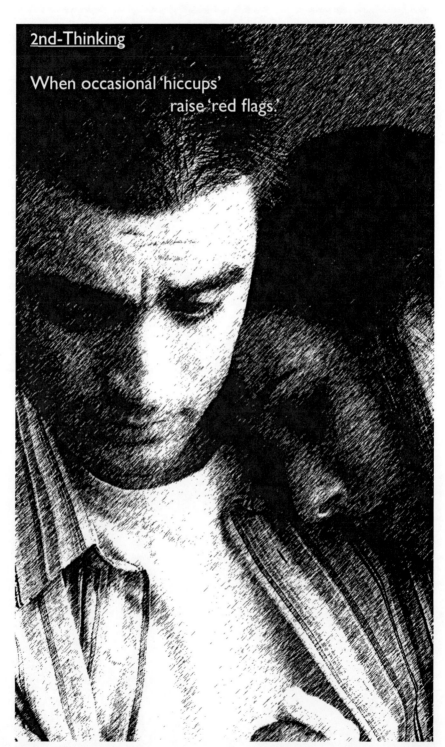

2nd-Thinking

When occasional 'hiccups'
                    raise 'red flags.'

<u>"Second thoughts"</u> ...

... are commonplace among Couples, both before and long after wedding ceremonies take place. Or if they never marry, too.

Bridal showers help assuage "wedding jitters." ("Wow — look what we got; all this new stuff!")

Bachelorette and classic Bachelor Parties help get the Bride- and Groom-to-be through, too. ("Don't think — just enjoy ... then do it!")

There are many, many situations, however, that can trigger feelings of unease.

Something could be said or done (or not said, not done) by your 'C'-mate, a friend or relative or even complete "outsiders" regarding your relationship.

It may be a sudden,
unexpected outburst or a routine mannerism you haven't noticed before.

Or maybe you're feeling neglected — taken for granted. Or perhaps, (dare I say it?) ... bored.

'Annoying mannerism?'

Or

'Endearing Trait?'

Sometimes there's a very fine line between the two.

What's more, where that line is drawn may simply be a matter of (as the saying goes) "which side of the bed you got up on today."

In short, "don't sweat the small stuff." (At least not too much.)

When hiccups occur ...

... you probably will find yourself wondering "Is this what's in store ...?" "Can it be altered or eliminated?" And if not, "Can I live with it?"

Many factors could influence how you proceed. First things first, however:

Pay attention

Don't ignore or totally shrug off "little voices" when they tell you that something doesn't seem right. At least delve into it far enough in your own mind — or discuss it with someone who may be familiar with the situation.

Then see if it merits a closer look, or no more concern.

Don't panic

Fact is, most "hiccups" need not be "relationship killers" at all. Bring it up, discuss it together and chances are, corrective action or a mutually acceptable compromise can happen in short order. More than that, remember:

> Hiccups are part of Life ... a
> naturally occurring, inevitable part.

Simply dealing with them — uncomfortable or annoying as they sometimes can be — helps to strengthen your bonds as a Couple. Which in turn, makes it easier to resolve future issues that arise.

"Drink water out of the 'wrong side' of the glass."

Maybe "Couple's Hiccups" can be resolved by learning from techniques used when people physically "get the hiccups." These hiccups also can occur anytime.

The water technique (above) from a 'C'-mate of mine calls for tipping the glass <u>away</u> from you, rather than toward you. This, then, requires you to extend your head and neck forward — over the closer (higher) edge of the glass … in order to sip without the water spilling.

The angle and extra effort do the trick.

<u>Lesson for Couples</u>:

Try looking at your hiccup from another angle — in a different way (or two or three ways). A little extra effort helps, too. Fresh perspectives often reveal things you haven't seen before. And that can open new avenues for resolution.

"Eat
a spoonful of sugar."

It may be an "old wives tale" and "a spoonful of sugar helps the medicine go down" was long-ago memorialized in song. Fact is: it works. A teaspoonful of plain ol' sugar — maybe because it tastes so good (and disrupts throat-air patterns or …?) Who cares? It gets rid of hiccups.

Obvious lesson for Couples: Be nice.

Calm, clear discussion easily beats being angry or upset (or "the silent treatment"). Every time.

Something may trigger ...

... an argument that starts with a "specific" (whatever was said or done) which can easily spread into much broader areas and issues.

That's good ... in the sense of uncovering problems that can never be solved until you know what they are.

That's bad — if the two of you are simply getting into a shouting match ... maybe making ancillary (but irrelevant) comments and accusations, and ...

> ... most of all,
> It's bad if you're not really _Listening_.

Earlier I noted that "Listening is the first half of talking. Actually, it's more like 90%."

Believe it. Act upon it. When your 'C'-mate speaks, shut up and listen. Really listen. Maybe repeat some of what he or she says — to ensure that you heard correctly and understand.

Your time to speak will come.

The result is "Communicating." And that's what makes any Couple relationship work.

In the process, keep in mind "a spoonful of sugar," too.

"I'm not always right.

*But I'm
very seldom wrong!"*

Said with a smile, often accompanied by a laugh, these words can work wonders. I've seen (actually, "heard") it happen.

See for yourself: Next time you and your 'C'-mate "share different opinions" ... try it!

Hopefully, whatever the issue is, you'll be able to put it behind you.

Dwelling on the past makes it difficult to look ahead.

Which, in turn, makes it impossible to find the future you want.

A simple (yet crucial) suggestion ...

<u>*forgive ... forget*</u>

"It happened once again today.
It hurt me and I turned away
from feelings warm and tender ...
If this is 'us' — why bother?"

"I hear you, Love. And I hurt, too.
No way I meant to make you cry.
No way I want to say good-by."

"Talk to me. Tell me true.
Where's an answer for we two?"

"Share our thoughts,
        clear our view
            ... act on what we see."

The answer comes from
you and me ...

Can we forgive?
Can we forget?
Find that Love's not over yet?
After all that we've been through
there's still a place for me 'n you.

It's in our hearts when we
forgive ... forget.

Putting your finger on …

… whatever is bothersome can prove to be an elusive pursuit —
yet vital to getting over the "speed bumps" you and your 'C'-mate
have encountered.

It's easy to say "we drifted apart." It's also a cop-out, and does
nothing to help you — individually, or as a couple.

So … continue to question, to pursue answers and reasons why.
Don't get so caught up in this, however, that your life & times
together become a constant search for imperfections. You will
no doubt find them. (A self-fulfilling prophecy.)

> Shifting your focus into positive-forward gear can,
> in and of itself, ease irritations that you've felt (but
> haven't identified).

You may even find yourself saying "Wow — this is good! Much
better than (whatever)." … And Presto! Suddenly you have
identified an issue <u>and</u> a way to resolve it.

Remember, too, that "every little thing" need not require detailed
reasons-why analysis. If one of you doesn't like something that
the other has a habit of doing, chances are you can just agree to
stop doing it. Period. Problem solved.

Friends 'n Family ...

... can often provide valuable insights — just as they did earlier when you and your 'C'-mate were getting to know each other.

Now, however, you're more likely to turn to your own close friends or relatives. But don't exclude his/hers, if you have developed a good communicative relationship with them.

Furthermore, any conversations between you need not be couched in terms of "we have a problem." I know of situations in which girl-talk as well as guy-talk about 'C'-mates revealed previously undetected factors contributing to issues, as well as unsolicited opinions.

> _"I love him to pieces,_
> _but I couldn't_
> _live with that man."_

Former girlfriends/boyfriends of your 'C'-mate, brothers and sisters or in-laws may provide perspectives that confirm "2nd thoughts" that you're having or, conversely, ease your mind.

You may discover things that <u>you</u> can do (or avoid) all by yourself that will ease the discomfort between you.

More likely, you'll glean nuggets of info and identify items to bring up with your 'C'-mate. Often you can simply allude to an event or issue from the past — which gets him or her started and enlightens both of you, considerably.

Realize, of course, that insights are only as good as what you do with them.

Can partners really change?

Do we really want them to?

("… Until tweaks do us part …")

For better or for worse ...

Can you and/or your 'C'-mate change? You bet. In many ways which make a major difference in your Couple-ship.

When you care, you try; you do your best to please.

Sometimes — Wow! — a few little tweaks ease the tensions and help reawaken the magic. I know it can.

For you? For me? How about "for Us"?

While it's nice to make changes to please your partner, ideally both of you will find them changes for the better.

A new hair style. Shaving a beard. Contemporizing one's wardrobe. Taking dance lessons. Trying a new-to-one, familiar to the other card game. Being less picky about how tasks are done — in the kitchen, out in the yard, whatever or wherever. Make your own list. It'll be fun.

Beware how far you push, however. It could ultimately backfire. To paraphrase the traditional wedding ceremony
... "until tweaks do us part."

There's also a surefire winner — to me, worth repeating — that virtually all Couples would do well to remember:

Listening better.

More closely. More attentively. More singularly focused. (Remember "moments" mentioned in "Getting to know you"?) Listening without multitasking … and without formulating your response until <u>after</u> your partner is done.

Despite all of this, sometimes changes don't seem to help — or have a very temporary impact. This can make the efforts seem even more frustrating. And also indicate that you *haven't yet uncovered the real issues at all.*

The uphill struggle down

I have never been so lonely in my life
than living here with you, dear,
as my wife.
    The more I show my love for you,
    the less you seem to want me to.
I have never been so lonely
in my life.

You used to say my working late
    was one thing wrong …
that your days were harder, too,
    'til I came home.
    So I've tried — with much success
    — to give us more togetherness.
But I've never been so lonely
in my life.

I'm too intense, you've said, which
    often spoils your mood.
I should relax — and things will happen
    as they should.
    But my quiet tenderness
    seems to do no good, I guess,
'cause I've never been so lonely
in my life.

You've also said I try too hard
    to "get things done."
We need to find more ways to
    simply have some fun.

While our social life's increased,
  making love has all but ceased.
I have never been so lonely in my life.

You want more freedom to pursue
    your own career ...
chances to do things "for yourself";
    and I concur.
Though "being out" first fed your fires,
now it dampens your desires.
I have never been so lonely in my life.

Years ago I worked much longer hours
    — and how!
I gave less for love from others
    than right now.
    But I never felt the way
    that I do now, night and day.
I have never been so lonely in my life.

I have never been so lonely in my life
than living here with you, dear,
as my wife.
    The more I show my love for you,
    the less you seem to want me to.
I have never been so lonely
in my life.

"Signs" & signposts

Ever had your fortune told? Some folks follow daily horoscopes, seek palm readings, use tarot cards, and gaze into crystal balls religiously (so to speak).

And if they sense discomfort in their 'C'-mate relationship, more than ever they're likely to seek such "insights" in order to:

- assuage (or confirm) their fears
- uncover problems or root causes of them
- find other reasons to rationalize feelings
- guide their moves.

Most of the time (in my view), horoscopes are nebulous statements — more fun to read at the end of the day ("Oh ... maybe that's why this-or-that happened ...").

And every once in awhile, they hit home.

Horrorscope

There the newspaper lies,
piercing through my eyes,
filling my head
    with dread.
I don't like what I see.
Does it really mean me?
I wish that I
    were dead.

    Horrorscope!
    Tells me you'll be gone.
    Horrorscope!
    Says I'll be alone.
    Horrorscope!
    Is there any other way?
      Maybe
    it's just for today …

My heart starts to bleed.
I continue to read:
"You'll find much
    happiness."
It describes who he'll be
and it doesn't sound like me!
Can't fight the fates,
    I guess.

    Horrorscope!
    Tells me you'll be gone.
    Horrorscope!
    Says I'll be alone.
    Horrorscope!
    Is there any other way?
      Maybe
    it's just for today …

© RES[4]

149

Sex (or lack thereof) ...

... frequently is a lightning rod when contemplating problems among Couples.

Too often, that's too easy an answer. And in some cases (maybe many), it's simply not true.

I know of one woman who professed having "great sex" with her husband. I also know that he agreed. Yet they are now "ex" husband and wife.

Fact is, sexual gratification is only part of any Couple's life. Other aspects of your relationship are even more crucial — while also (directly or indirectly) affecting sexual activity and your satisfaction from it.

It's also a fact that sex (or the lack thereof) can trigger a two-step pull-apart process: one partner is driven away and, sooner or later, either or both partners are drawn to someone else.

Before it's too late, let your 'C'-mate know that you sense a problem here. Try to pinpoint what's behind it — and what you as a Couple can do about it.

> Face it: You and your 'C'-mate
> are a living, breathing entity. Life
> is a process in constant change.

The trick is to "change for the better."

That will never happen, however, unless and until you let him or her know what you think, how you feel …

Love me stay

Nothing here for me
but another lonely night.
    You're too tired,
    don't feel well or
something's just not "right."
    No need to lay
    with you in our bed.
    Might as well stay
somewhere else instead.

You say that you love me
more as time goes on,
    but you just can't
    waken passion
when the day is done.
    Emptiness reigns
    with you in our bed.
    Is fuller love
somewhere else instead?

It's not that I want
to seek another's arms.
    But with workday
    battles done,
I long for soothing charms
    … your warmth
    surrounding me in our bed.
    Maybe there's warmth
somewhere else instead.

Nothing here for me;
yet everything could be.
    Can't you see?
    No one else
has aroused such fires in me!
    Love … don't just lay
    with me in our bed,
    lest I should stray
somewhere else instead.

"Little white lies" …

or maybe simply telling less than "the whole truth" often seems like a good idea if you (or your 'C'-mate) become involved with someone else.

The usual rationale is that you don't want to hurt your current partner.

Think again.

Sooner or later, somehow your affair will be found out.

It's not a question of "if." It's merely a matter of "when."

And chances are, long before that happens, your partner will sense that something's going on.

He or she may not want to say anything. (After all, if you can't _trust_ your 'C'-mate, who can you …?)

As for "hurting" your partner:

I can tell you firsthand that the Agony of Suspecting can pierce far deeper than wielding the Sword of Truth.

Another Night

Lying in bed
    alone,
waiting for you.
Wondering where
    you've gone.
Wondering who

… is making you
smile tonight,
feeling your love?
    All I can do
    is watch
the cold moon above.

    Another night,
    hating your lies.
    Another night —
    my heart slowly dies.
        I can't
        breathe!
    The pain hurts me so.
    The emptiness
    flows and covers
    my soul.

You may find yourself ...

... making lists as you feel your 'C'-mate slipping away. It's not unlike list-making when finding your 'C'-mate.

Only now, instead of listing "what I want" in a partner, your list consists of "what we've got" as a Couple (e.g. financial stability, great sex, opportunities to travel ...)

Plusses and minuses put on paper can be an excellent step toward clarifying your own thoughts. As you list "items," you'll also realize other, more-emotional aspects that may affect the way you and/or your partner feel.

Sharing lists, if nothing else, tells him or her that you're concerned, that you care and that you want to do something about it.

This also could help you begin working together (after all, you are a Couple) to isolate specific problems ... and collaborate on finding ways to solve them.

Sometimes a partner may use plus-and-minus lists to try convincing the other partner that they're best off staying together because they have "so much going" for them.

Good luck. Such list-sharing may help either or both of you to stop and think a bit.

But the Logic of Lists seldom trumps the "Feelings Card."

Outside help ...

... in the form of counseling often can direct Couples toward those deeper, hidden root causes of problems.

Provided, of course, both partners are willing and open to pursue and probe their issues in such a venue.

Individual as well as joint sessions encourage parties to speak more openly and directly.

You can learn a lot. About yourself, first of all, as well as about your 'C'-mate, your relationships with him or her and with other people in your life to-date.

The more you learn, the better you're able to find and take next steps — to get your relationship back on track.

I know of several Couples with whom this was the case; they did precisely that.

I also know Couples who learned something equally valuable, if not as pleasantly so. To wit:

That continuing their Couple-ship was NOT best for them.

'Another woman?'
'Another man?'

The ultimate issue
regarding your relationship
still lies between
your 'C'-mate and you.

Are you and he or she
as a 'We'
really meant to be?

Commission? Or Omission?

Whether or not your 'C'-mate has become involved with someone else, the more you think about life between you, the more you may start to see "little things" that add up big.

You may remember, for instance, his or her voice on the phone ...

> "I miss you so much!"

> "I want you — can't wait to see you."

> "I so much love having you here."

> "Can't wait for us to be together more than just weekends or several days at a time."

Have you heard those words lately? At all? Much less spoken with such passion?

You're probably not the only one.

What next? Of course, trying to find out "why" and "fix" whatever it is has to be Priority One. And I hope you'll be able to do so. Rest assured, however, that

"Life moves in Forward Motion." You can never go back.

Is it possible, however, to hold the Future at bay ...?

Hurry, Tomorrow

Hurry, Tomorrow ...
    (tomorrow, tomorrow)
Please don't ever come!

Hurry, Tomorrow ...
    (hurry, hurry)
so I can send you away ...!

    Loving you today
    will go on forever,
    if Tomorrow
    will only stay away.

    Love will be our future
    if Today won't leave us.
    I love you
    Today — ! Stay ...
            Stay ...

Hurry, Tomorrow ...
    (tomorrow, tomorrow)
Please don't ever come!

Hurry, Tomorrow ...
    (hurry, hurry)
so I can send you away ...!

160

Maybe someone comes along ...

... who seems to be the perfect match for your current (or hoped-for) 'C'-mate. You may know of such a case or two; I certainly do.

Remember the woman who met a man with "everything on her list"? (See "Finding your 'C'-mate.") The dude had megabucks, was a superb golfer, gourmet cook, DIY fix-it whiz ...

How does one compete with that?

You don't. And you don't have to.

> *True Love*
> *is not*
> *a contest.*

What makes Love real, is how you feel.

Surface trappings are merely that. No more, no less. And, in fact, you could easily become "trapped." I don't mean trapped by them, per se ... in the sense of someone's wealth or other advantages "buying your love" (or even your allegiance).

There's no denying that wealth and time for leisure, however, can be extremely liberating. The simple fact is ...

*'Money
can't buy happiness.*

*But it sure can buy
opportunity!'*

"Second thoughts?" Let me add a Third ...

Regardless of how much (or little) wealth is involved, think beyond how you feel toward your current C-mate or potential new mates. Think about how they feel towards you.

And I don't mean do they say, "I love you."

Rather ... Do they trust you?

Do they trust you to be your own person? ... To think your own thoughts? Do they trust you to feel however you wish to feel about others in your life?

More than that, are they at ease with your _right to feel and act on your own,_ as you wish? Or do they try to restrict (or even deny) your freedom to enjoy relationships?

Having a partner who's a bit jealous or protective isn't necessarily bad; in one sense, it's flattering.

If, however, that means restricting or denying your right to not only associate — but also your right to "feel for" someone else, and to act (however you choose) on your feelings ... very serious "2nd Thoughts" may be called for.

You see, to me, True Love does not prohibit or restrict:

True Love
sets
you Free.

Whatever your current or future
'C'-mate may provide,
remember:

'What you see
is what you get.'

*Is it really
what you want?*

Gifted

You had everything
 you could want
(or so it seemed).

Luxury home, lavishly furnished.
Fashionable clothes — always
 in style.
Exquisite jewelry,
 trendy accessories.
Leisure and travel — thousands
 of miles.

A Lovely Dove
 in a Gilded Cage.
Living a dream
all of your days.

It didn't come easy!
… working hard
 in tandem with
the love-of-your-life mate.
And there were "hiccups"
 along the way.
Yet, all in all,
 life was great.

Then
suddenly pushed
from the Gilded Cage,
    your life
turned upside-down.
Bewildered,
you found yourself in

            a free-fall

            toward

            the

            ground.

Head spinning, heart-sore,
total emptiness inside.
Devastated by rejection,
... and damage to your pride.

Yes, money would come
    to ensure a life of ease.
But it can't replace
dashed hopes and dreams
— worse than that:
        lost self-esteem.

A Lovely Dove
        from a Gilded Cage.
Losing your dream
in a foggy haze.

*   *   *   *

Then Love anew
> beckons you,
and breathes Life from within.

A Kindred Spirit …
he speaks to your heart,
> enriches your mind,
excites your nights and more.

You feel stronger each day
> — up-up, away …!
With your soul-mate
> you can soar
> > forward, onward,
> — flying freely
higher than e'er before.

*   *   *   *

Now

comes a new bird;

wants to fly in tandem with you.

A perfect match

    for the life you like.

And quite charming, too.

Again you can have

    everything you want

(or so it seems):

Money, golf, gourmet touch,

fix-it skills and more;

furnishings, fashionings

    and traveling for you.

With the time

    and wherewithal

        to do it all, too.

A Lovely Dove,

      new Gilded Cage.

Is this the dream

for the rest of your days?

Perhaps

it's what you want.

Perhaps it's what you need.

Perhaps

I'd best keep silent

... accept your destiny.

But questions, Love,

    keep haunting me ...

Does he seek to limit

times you spend

    with others close to you?

Or try to deny

    your *Freedom to Feel?*

Does he not "trust"

what you might do?

Does he say he cares

— that's why he needs to

    shield your life from harm?

Clipping your wings

while giving you things ...

Will it keep you safe

        and warm?

"You dare not fly free.

　　　You belong to me."

Is this his message, in effect?

Are you,

to him, merely a new

　　　possession he must protect?

Lovely Dove

　in a Gilded Cage ...

I fear not

a full, rich life for you

— days of smiles and fun.

I fear for your heart,

your soul ... true freedom

　　for your dreams ...

　and a lingering emptiness inside,

when those days are done.

You see,

it may be new,

more gilded, too

... filled with exquisite things.

Yet I fear

his love,

My Dove,

returns you

to a cage.

My Love

gives you Wings ...

"But - but you

always liked that

before ..."

You can sense ...

... what's going on in your 'C'-mate's heart and mind.

It's one of the more wonderful aspects of the life to-date you've enjoyed together.

It's also the most awful

      ... when that heart-sinking feeling tells you that Un-Coupling is about to begin.

Chapter 6

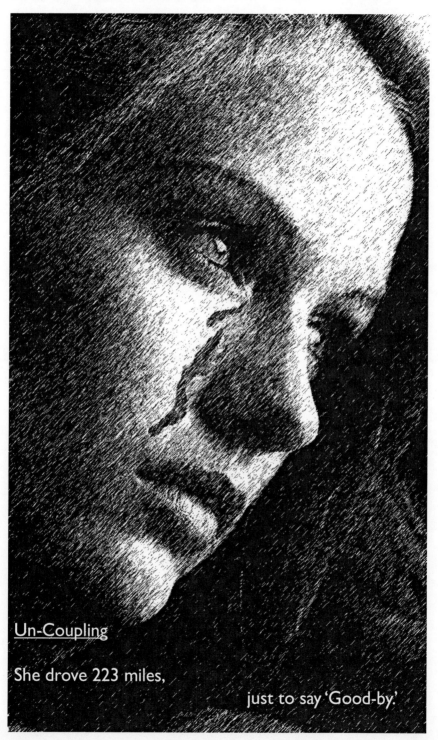

Un-Coupling

She drove 223 miles,

just to say 'Good-by.'

Tears rolled slowly

… down her cheeks and in-between sobs, she said

"I love you."   Also …

"It isn't you — it's me."
"I need time."
"I need space."
"I need room to breathe."
   And the inevitable,
"I don't want to hurt you."

'Kisses of death,'
I call them. One or more presage virtually every Un-Coupling.
Guaranteed. And this time, I heard them all. I was, if you will,
"smothered with 'Kisses.'"

Over the years, enough Couplings (and Un-Couplings) have enriched my life to recognize the signs. All too quickly. And, yes, I said "enriched." I cherish every one; and every "Un-."

In addition to less formal relationships, I've had enough fiancées to be able to refer to them as "my first fiancée, my last fiancée, the fiancée I married" ... and I have too-often heard the <u>sequel</u> to "Kisses of death":

"Marrying me wouldn't be right for you."
Or "Living together ..." or "Being with me ..." or a variation pertinent to our particular Couple situation.

In any case, you've gotta love how they always say that this is best for you. And how much it hurts them.

All of which, I believe, ultimately is true. Nevertheless ...

> *Your eyes cry ... My heart bleeds.*

Backing off from

… a relationship is almost always a gut-wrenching affair.
For both parties.

Especially if you really care, yet feel that a permanent alliance isn't what you want. It's also tough, however, when discontent has been obvious for some time.

In any case, take a lesson from a lyric (not written by me):

"A little kindness sure might help mend a broken heart."*

Kindness … compassion … genuine concern are crucial. And that applies to both parties — the one <u>receiving</u> the bad news, as well as the 'C'-mate conveying it.

More than ever, these are moments in which to respect each other — what you've had, where you are and, as best you can communicate it, where and what you want to be.

It doesn't hurt, of course, to try to dissuade your 'C'-mate, or to alter his/her decision. In fact, if you truly care and feel a viable future as a Couple still exists, by all means — give it a go.

Realize, however, that — like the business person who resigns a position, then is persuaded to stay — odds are good that the "reconsidered" action will be of short duration.

Ultimately, if you're on the receiving end of "good-by," you can simply say "OK," and disappear. You may, however, feel moved to say a bit more. For example …

What do you say

… to the One you've loved
and lived for, be it a few months
or many years?

What do you say
when they say they need space
— and can't live with you anymore?

You say
"Thanks."
Thanks for the memories wherever I look,
and a multitude more locked in my mind.
"Thanks …"
For the warm days
in your sun, for the times that were such fun.
For the offspring
only we could bear; so much that's ours alone
to share.
"Thanks…"
For a world of new beginnings. Yes, even
the future we face now …

After all, if your relationship bore nothing
for which to be thankful — and from which
to grow, what's the point?
<RES>

© RES[4] (adapted)

Maybe you're the one ...

... who decided it was time to Un-Couple.

As the saying goes,

> _"It's a rotten job — but somebody's got to do it."_

Whatever the reason (probably several), hopefully you'll be honest and straightforward — and kind enough — to not "burn bridges" between you and your now-former 'C'-mate.

Not just because you don't want to hurt him or her. But also because, for one, the future could still hold pleasant times for the two of you. (See "Post-Couple Coupling.")

Certainly if you are (or were) married with children, you could (and, I hope, would) share custody and child-rearing duties. I can also vouch for enjoying times with kids and a former spouse after your children are "all grown up."

And, believe it or not, the two of you may one day get back together — on a less- or more-permanent basis than before.

You never know.

Meanwhile, for now ... Any regrets ...?

Lib Lady

Why the tear, my Dear?
… a tugging unrelenting,
   rending your facade.
   Everyone knows
Liberated Ladies don't weep.

Is it business pressures?
Social doldrums?
   No. And even so,
neither "Cosmo" nor the
tabloids can relate to what you
know:

That *once you lost (or by-passed)*
   a once-per-lifetime mate.
And an emptiness inside
says perhaps it wasn't wise
   to have messed with fate.

So shed that tear, my Dear.
   Let it flow unrelenting,
   rending your facade.
   Let the world know
Liberated Ladies can weep …

And if you're not ...

... the initiator of the Un-Coupling, it can drive you nuts trying to figure out "why — what's behind this?"

Your departed (or departing) 'C'-mate may, in word or deed, give you a clue.

And no doubt, you'll have an inkling or two.

Little by little, the more you look, the more possibilities you'll see, the more answers you'll find.

Sometimes, in surprising places ...

The Other Woman

I'm sitting here, stunned.
You just walked out the door
and you didn't look back.
Never left like this before.

After years together,
after all I have done,
how could someone else
make you leave me alone?

"The other woman."
I must find who she is.
"The other woman"
who left me here like this.

Who could make you go
taking your love with you?
Is she beautiful?
But you said you were true!

Who could change your mind?
Who would do this to me?
I have all you want,
you kept telling me.

"The other woman."
I'll meet her, then I'll know.
"The other woman."
The one who made you go.

Will she soon find your
caresses leave her cool?
When you work late, will she
wonder who's with you?

Will she learn your love
buys nothing in a store?
Will she become me ...
'til you walk out the door?

"The other woman."
Suddenly I see her.
"The other woman"
is here ... in the mirror.
... in the mirror.

Certainly there's a gap

… in your life when someone with whom you're shared so much, now shares no more.

Often, however, there's little time to think about it.

For example, a woman I know who'd been living in Europe with her long-time husband (an exec, transferred by his company) … returned from a week-long fun-filled vacation with him at a French resort — and suddenly heard him say he wanted a divorce. Now.

Then he left to spend a week or so with his Mistress, leaving her to figure out where, when and how to move back to the States.

Brutal. Absolutely brutal.

In another situation, a husband suddenly found himself to be the "custodial parent" for kids still in school … with added responsibilities leaving little or no time to "think about it," either.

In this case, his now-former spouse was seeing another man, but the affair wasn't the "cause." She said she'd simply been "unhappy for years," married to him; and wanted "out."

Which prompts the question …

Which hurts worse:

- When your 'C'-mate leaves you for someone else?
- Or when your 'C'-mate simply leaves you?

If anyone can answer that, I suppose it would be me. I've been left both ways, more than once, each. (Ouch!) And one time, both at once — with the very same woman! (?... Understand? I'm not sure I do ...)

Whatever ... if they leave for someone else, realize that "losing" to someone else doesn't make you a "loser." Besides, it's only one game (so to speak).

Simply remind yourself that, in truth, it's his or her loss — not yours. You're OK, and on your way to finding someone new.

Nevertheless,
even if the two of you reach the point at which you "don't much like each other" anymore ... it still leaves a "gap" when you split.

You'll probably feel rather "drained" and weak; both mad and glad; sad, too. You'll hurt inside. You name it — chances are, you'll feel it ... along with other things you're not able to name.

All of which can be summed up in five letters:

E – M – P – T – Y

No burden's heavier ...

You walked into my world
when I was fancy-free.
You showed me how to Love,
and share it blissfully.

Then, swiftly as you came,
I woke and you were gone.
Though friends still think
    that I'm the same,
I don't feel very strong.

    ... 'cause I'm carrying
    the mem'ry of your charms.
    No burden's heavier
        than empty arms.

Before you came to me,
my life was just a breeze.
    And with you,
I still made my way
    with utmost ease.

My Love grew so!
'Twould last forever and a day.
Now Love still grows ... and
    grows ... and grows.
But you have gone away.

    ... and I'm carrying
    the mem'ry of your charms.
    No burden's heavier
        than empty arms.

No burden's heavier
... than
    empty
    arms.

Is there any such thing as ...

... a good "season" for Un-Coupling? In my view: Never.

I suppose some could be better or worse than others.

Christmas holidays come to mind. Everyone is partying with loved ones, enjoying family 'n friends get-togethers. And your usual New Year's Eve companion is ... where?

The good news is that you're off the hook on buying him or her Christmas gifts!

Once upon a time I used to joke about breaking up with partners just before Thanksgiving — then getting back together around February 15th. No Holiday gifts. No expensive New Year's dine 'n dance. No Valentine hearts 'n flowers.

That may be a way to save money; but it's not really funny and, in truth, those are some of the best times to enjoy with someone for whom you truly care.

Bad as you may feel, don't be afraid to spread the word about your Couple-ship's demise. With news of your availability, some of those Holiday venues could help jump-start your move to someone new and even better.

Every other season offers opportunities, too.

Summer – Fall – Winter – Spring ... perhaps the worst season in which to break up would be the season in which you met or, if you will, became a twosome.

189

One way to keep warm

Frost sparkled in the moonlight
    the night that we first met.
Nights grew longer.
Love grew stronger.
How can you forget?

You said you had to leave me
    with Winter setting in.
I yearned for Spring to spread its
wing, still hoping you'd return.

   Why'd you have to leave now?
   Couldn't you give us Spring?
   Why did you go to him?
   Does our Love mean nothing?

   I guess you always loved him,
   and that you meant no harm.
   You're married now, in Winter

   ... that's one way
      to keep warm.

You said "don't try to reach me";
that once you're gone, it's done.
But I couldn't make myself
believe I'd never be the One.

Now shattered hopes surround me
   since my phone call to you.

My full heart broke
as your voice spoke — although,
deep down I knew ...

   Why'd you have to leave now?
   Couldn't you give us Spring?
   Why did you go to him?
   Does our Love mean nothing?

   I guess you always loved him,
   and that you meant no harm.
   You're married now, in Winter

   ... that's one way
     to keep warm.

   You're married now, in Winter

   ... that's one way
     to keep warm.

Ultimate Un-Coupling

Standing just inside the guest room, she wrapped her arms around me and fused our still-clothed bodies tightly together.

I could feel her breasts ... her flat, firm stomach ... her hips and thighs melding with mine through the fabric as her lips drew us into a long, lingering passionate kiss.

"I love you," she murmured breathlessly, without allowing our lips to lose touch.

"And making love with you is the most phenomenal experience of all."

Our embrace intensified along the entire length of our bodies for several seconds longer.

Slowly, she withdrew her lips.
She smiled into my eyes.
Her fingertips lingered in my hand ever-so briefly
as she turned away.

Then she walked into the Master bedroom
            ... to him.

Even if...

... your departing 'C'-mate is not currently involved with another partner, you can bet that sooner or later he or she will be.

There's nothing you can do about it.

They win — You lose.

Except, in one respect, maybe not ...

avant-garde heart

It's no surprise to me
that men keep calling you.
Your smile
brings on the sunshine.
Your lips glisten like dew.
And when your eyes
        sparkle so bright
— none can resist you then.
But though they're with you
        and I'm not,
I'm ahead of other men.

    Let them fall in love with you.
    I know chapter and verse,
    how you'll break
    their hearts in two.
    'cause you broke my heart first.

Men love to feel your hair
fall rich and golden down
… your silky-smooth caresses,
your soft skin tanned so brown.
And when you whisper
        "come to me"
they can't turn back again.
But though they rush
        into your arms,
I'm ahead of other men.

    Let them fall in love with you.
    I know chapter and verse,
    how you'll break
    their hearts in two
    'cause you broke my heart first.

© RES

194

If being the first ...

... to have your heart broken doesn't give you much comfort (and I can see why it wouldn't),

> _Take heart._
> (yes, I said "heart")

There's still hope. And it may be closer than you think.

Just around the corner

No matter how it seems,
hold onto your dreams.
      Look up
to the voice that says
      somehow
your spirit will outrun
dark clouds and find
      the sun!

Just around the corner
   from right now.

No matter where you are
reach out for your star.
    It's yours.
And your dreams
will show you how
you can rise up and soar
higher than e'er before!

Just around the corner
   from right now.

Can you not feel it
in the air?
Winds whisper
"Destiny draws near."
Dreams carry you there
and they'll come true
for you there …!

No matter how it seems,
hold onto your dreams.
Look up.
Heed the voice that says
somehow
your spirit will outrun
dark clouds and find
the sun!

Just around the corner
from right now.

Just around the corner
from right now.

A positive outlook ...

... not only puts your mind into feel-good mode, it also enhances your chances of attracting a new (maybe "The") 'C'-mate.

Telling yourself things are good, of course, doesn't make them that way.

And now and then, you'll still think back ... and remember "the end" ...

That morning ...

... we reversed our usual roles.

You put on the coffee
     and I made breakfast:
  French toast (with Italian bread),
  jumbo eggs scrambled
     with cheddar,
  mini-sausage nibblets and
  tomato juice with a dash
     of Worcestershire and
     Tabasco, topped
     with a sprinkle of pepper.
  Plus banana nuggets,
  neatly sliced by you.

We've enjoyed many breakfasts & brunches, and today's was no exception. Yet for me, at least, the dreams I wanted to hold onto seemed to not be "just around the corner." In fact, no "corner" was in sight.

As I said one time, regarding Us and your divorce: "The hopes and dreams you had, were shattered. And I didn't have any, until You ... and We."

Thank you for that. For every single hope, every single dream.

What will they now become? I haven't a clue.

As for Us, before we ever talked last night, I knew ...

last lover

Swiftly flees the twilight
— I see it in your eyes.

A world anew
   beckons you
      onward to sunrise.

But first,
one more remembrance:
      a night
     of nights

… to calm your fears,
   to dry your tears,
and tell you it's all right.

No philanderer, I.
You are my One.

Were once we first for each?
More than then?
And again?

I suppose it matters not,
on this day's Only night
   as time runs on
and darkening shadows
overtake the light.

New mysteries will arise
to greet you with the dawn.

No need to fear;
come to me here
… again tonight you'll find
    inner peace
as you gather strength
before our time is gone

            and you move on,
    leaving Us
behind.

I feel you surround me,
    sense your desire,
equal your passion
— hot flowing fire.

Thank you for caring,
for sharing with me.
    For Us,
these brief moments
a lifetime shall be.

Chapter 7

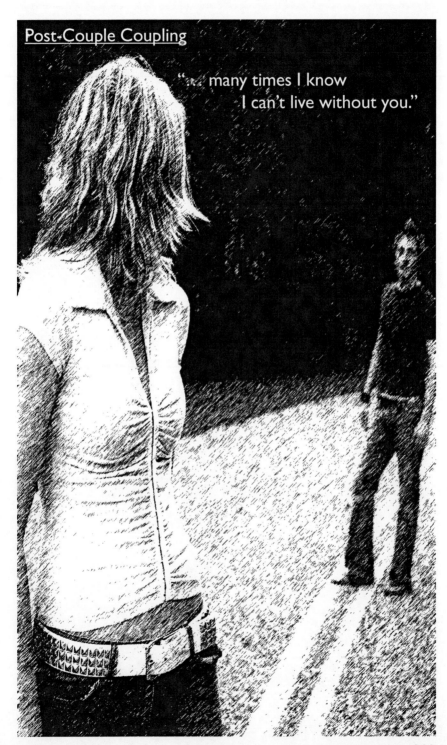

All too often

… Un-Coupling is presumed to mean "ending" the relationship. Totally. Completely. Good-by — you are now out of my life.

Certainly that's wise when abusive or destructive behavior is a factor. Sometimes for other reasons, too.

I submit, however, that most Couples have gained much from each other … forming a foundation upon which they can build and with which they can continue to grow, individually and, perhaps, even as a twosome.

An old adage, "Don't throw out the baby with the bathwater" comes to mind. Why let positive things that the two of you achieved, still enjoy and appreciate, go to waste?

Despite Un-Coupling, you and your former 'C'-mate more than likely find some things about or with each other that you really-really don't want to lose.

"Many times I know I can't live without you."

There is no need to.

True, you may no longer see each other every day, make love every night (did you "back then"?) or plan your lives as a twosome.

I contend, however, that you and your former 'C'-mate can continue to give each other key things that made your relationship so special in the first place.

It merely calls for a bit of advanced Couple-ship thinking.

Apart-ners

It pains me sometimes
to see us apart,
   although I know
   it's for the best,
deep down in my heart.

Yet, no other can match
the comfort you bring
... the joy and the wonder
   in so many ways
   on so many days ...
And it doesn't need a ring
on your finger ...
        Just you.

Your voice o'er the phone.
A visit. A smile.
Your ear — just to hear
me talk for a while.

It's not much to ask.
It's not much to give.
And it means that you care,
in truth, how I live.

Separately we can grow,
encouraging each other
     as we go.
It's a new, special love
from deep in our heart,
as we travel new roads
    together apart.

© RES

206

Growing together apart,

… isn't at all as difficult or unusual as it may at first seem.

To be sure, the party who did <u>not</u> initiate Un-Coupling could find continued contact more painful than helpful — at least at first blush. After all …

Healing from heartbreak, like life itself, is a process.

I know the drill. All too well.

I also can assure you that the together-apart concept can help you not only take a step in that process, but find a road to wherever you want to be.

> _"I think of you a lot._
> _And I think_
> _a lot of you."_

The idea is to move forward, drawing strength and support from every worthy source. And your former 'C'-mate just could be one of the most worthy, ever.

*"The essence of what we have
hasn't changed."*

*"No matter what
happens down the line,
there is no one
that I would
feel closer to than you."*

You may find ...

(as I have) that <u>looking ahead</u> often comes easier — and the new view gets clearer — when you spend a little time looking back.

Not wallowing in self-pity, mind you, but recalling times (good and bad) and <u>thinking</u> about what those recollections bring to you now ... and to where you want to be.

When it comes to looking ahead by looking back ...

There's a lot to be said

... for pictures. Photographs. Snapshots.

I take tons, chronicling Life as it's lived. Candidly. On-the-fly.
People, places, pets, events ... Life. Captured on 35 mm film.
Including times with 'C'-mates.

Of course, in these Digital days, telephones also function as
cameras. Computer users can scan and upload, download ...
show friends 'n family the latest, almost as it happens.

Not so incidentally, a good deal of digital doctoring also
sometimes goes on ... combining or otherwise altering images to
project impressions that may be, shall we say, less than accurate.

Whatever, I ultimately find a stronger sense of reality in hard-copy photo prints. Good (and sometimes, bad) shots wind up in my photo albums.

Some people are both more selective and more elaborate ... scrap-booking photos with other memorabilia, too.

Either way — especially in Post-Couple life — I respectfully submit that clicking and scrolling on a computer screen to view pictures ...

in no way can match the breadth, depth, vividness — or the excitement and warmth of memories evoked with a photo album or scrapbook in-hand.

Hello, Yesterdays

Hello, Yesterdays.
It's nice to be with you
    in a photo album,
    flipping through.
You look just great
from where I sit.
      You know,
you haven't changed a bit!

Hello, Memories.
You warm me through
    and through.
Time has been so very
      kind to you.
Each page that I turn
adds so to your glow

… so thank you
for inviting me.
    Yesterdays,
    Hello …!

You'll notice things

… reminders of your times together. Everywhere.

Go ahead: look. It's a cleansing process. Yes, even when it hurts.

You'll find things your 'C'-mate left behind or, perhaps, brought back.

"You left the ring," I said o'er the phone, staring at the diamonds-in-platinum band specially designed to perfectly conform to the contours of the engagement ring she wore … no more.

"It doesn't go with anything I have," I added, half jokingly.

She replied, "It doesn't go with anything that I have, either."
Touche.

'I miss you. Terribly.'

*'But if We
hadn't been,*

*I'd have missed
a lot more.'*

Those tight, white ...

terry cloth shorts — remember them? *(See "Getting to know you,"* '*C*'-2.) Laundered. Neatly folded. Ready for another wearing that will never come.

And the socks. That pair I pulled from the drawer when she hadn't packed any, and her shoeless feet were cold despite (or maybe because of) the fever she was running.

She pulled on the socks and lay down on the couch, snuggled under an afghan and that soft, fresh-laundered earth-tone blanket that my cat loves so well. My cat even curled up on her lap.

Plus the on-the-rocks glass with my initials on it — the one from which she sipped her favorite Scotch.

In short, the two of you share a lot of history. You could share a future, too — albeit on somewhat different terms.

If your former 'C'-mate

…and you find common ground for continuing to see each other (and I hope you will, even if only now 'n then) many pleasant new times can enhance both of your lives.

Often, this takes the form of dating — "going out" to movies or other events; dinner, perhaps; or even showing up together at parties, as New Year's Eve partners and the like.

Sometimes, however, contact between you and your former 'C'-mate is also (or instead) less public — especially if you and he/she live near one another.

Then, stopping by for dinner … taking a walk in the park … picking up an outfit before the cleaner closes … sharing pizza and beer while watching "the big game" — all can provide pleasant interludes and comfortable companionship.

Sometimes one can repair a household item or show the other how to master a recipe or … you name it. Or you could assist your former 'C'-mate in more-subtle ways, even including new romantic pursuits.

Best of all, there's usually no "standing on ceremony" in a relationship like this.

You've known each other; been with each other. You have, in the past, seen each other "at your worst."

Time shared without pretenses is time to be cherished, indeed.

eye class

I've seen you
with your glasses on
    and loved your eyes
the more.

Yet I sensed dismay in your
voice at a simple little chore …
lighting the gas-log fireplace
    ("I'll need to put
    my glasses on …")
    on any given night
with a companion in sight.

(After all,
it could break the mood
as you and he
move toward intimacy
— that thought instantly
clicked with me.)

So I showed you how to
    light by touch,
with fingertips on the knob
… a smooth, swift
spectacles-free way
       to fire-up the log.

Now you're all set;
I'll soon be gone.
    Your vanity aside,
one thing's crystal-clear:

If at times, my Love,
glasses help you see,
there's no way that
    your beauty's lost
when your fireside lover's me.

"Last night ...

... we didn't make love.
     We loved.
Huddling beneath the covers,
combating the early Autumn chill.
     Together."

Sometimes, former 'C'-mate "sleepovers" occur. Not the hot, passionate sexual trysts of bygone days. But, "hey — it's late, we're both tired; spend the night."

Rather than the blanket-on-a-couch or guest room gambit, they may choose to (you guessed it) share the same bed.

When former 'C'-mates care deeply, they also recognize and respect that previous times are gone; that each is moving on. "Bedtime" means sleep, not sex.

Don't be surprised if hugs or even a goodnight kiss are part of the process, however. Many times I've slept with a beautiful woman in my arms all night, without making love.

It feels good. And I never really thought about "why." Then one night, a 'C'-mate phrased it exquisitely:

> *"If we never made love again*
> *and I held you in my arms,*
> *I would be complete."*

Wow. Me, too.

There's a sanctity in closely cradling one who is important to you. There's quiet comfort in your togetherness. And unspeakable peace when, in time, you drift off to sleep.

Whether or not you make love, the simple fact is ...

It's nice to share

'Good night'

with one you truly

care for.

And 'Good morning,' too.

Sometimes nothing ...

... transpires immediately or consistently with former 'C'-mates. And that's OK, too.

After all, each of you is moving on, and no rule says you need (or even want) to take parallel paths.

As time passes and individual Un-Coupled lives evolve, either or both parties may discover new perspectives on their past times together.

They may realize that things "weren't all that bad" or, even better, that their times together yielded deeper, more positive benefits.

One case comes to mind, which prompted a single but warmly memorable one-time visit.

Thanks

It's too late to come home.
I don't live here anymore.
But I had to see you
… tell you things
   I didn't know before.

Now my life is my own.
Now I'm able to see
   all the things you did
   to make it possible
for me to be me.

Is there sex

… in the Post-Couple era? Should there be? The obvious answer is … several answers.

Certainly if either or both parties are now Coupled with someone else, sexual relations is probably not a good idea. Probably a *bad* idea, in fact.

Beyond that … many former 'C'-mates date each other following divorce or other non-marital separation — often enjoying each other's company far more than when they lived together.

> *"We never had sex.*
> *But we sure did*
> *some great love-making."*

If they still find each other sexually desirable, compatible and choose to do so — why not? Occasional (or even frequent) trysts can be mutually satisfying in many ways.

"Listen to me,"
she said emphatically;
then paused.

("Yes? I'm listening.")

"I ... love ... you."
(Another pause.)

"I love
making love with you.
Big time.
And I absolutely love
how you
make love to me."

Perhaps there's a place

... for passionate and cozy-comfy rest stops along the road of life.

Realize, however, that sooner or later, your partner may lose interest — or move on to someone else.

Consider this warning from my past ...

'next time...'

Sunrise, the crack of dawn.
In seconds I'll be gone.
You turn and slumber on
    nestled in your flannel sheets.
Last night's
loving that we shared
...the touch beyond compare
told each the other cared
and made us feel complete

...until next time.
        Except...

"Next time" may be never
you reminded me
        last night.
"Next time" may be never
        though this time
        felt so right.
In you and me
you do not see
    a lifetime future "we."
"Next time" may be never.
    Our time
    was last night.

"Nothing's changed"
        you murmured.
The same is true for me.
While you see roads to
nowhere,
        I hope
        one leads to "we."

Or maybe there are rest stops
                    like this
          along the way
where (for a little while)
we hold the world
at bay

...until next time.
          And yet...

"Next time" may be never
you reminded me
          last night.
"Next time" may be never
          though this time
          felt so right.
In you and me
you do not see
     a lifetime future "we."
"Next time" may be never.
     Our time
     was last night.

"Nothing's changed"
          you murmured
despite your lips on mine
...and fingertips touching
skin so smooth, so fine.
"Nothing's changed"
          you murmured
and still our pleasure's real.
          "One more thing
before we sleep..."
how good you make me feel

...until next time.
          Except...

"Next time" may be never
you reminded me
     last night.
"Next time" may be never
     though this time
     felt so right.
In you and me
you do not see
     a lifetime future "we."
"Next time" may be never.
     Our time
     was last night.

     *   *   *   *

Sunrise, the crack of dawn
     with you and me and
     night now gone

when suddenly
     it occurs to me
     as I quietly slip out,
that nights like this
     and times
like ours
are what life's all about.

So "next time" may be never.
     And yet it also seems
"next times"
     may come for
          ever

on wings of hopes and dreams.

The secret ...

... to growing together apart _happily_, ultimately lies in managing expectations. Yours. And your former 'C'-mate's.

Openness and honesty — the kind you (hopefully) practiced when you were a Couple — still hold true.

And it ensures continuation of a mutually satisfying relationship.

Which, after all, is what Couples are all about.

...one night

Today began for us nearly 21 hours ago.
        But only a few have passed since
we held each other and I said
        I feared that this might
        frighten you away
 from me ... from us ....
        And you replied that
if we both want something
and maybe
it's merely a one night stand
— and if we can handle that ...

Suddenly once again,
            you turned the key
and unlocked the secret:

If one night for us
leads to many,
    each will still be

            one

... unique, special,
its own entity filled with
its own wonder
like no other, before or next ...

without comparison.

No expectations.
Pure acceptance.

Like relationships:
Remember when I said that everyone
(including us) has relationships
—but all too often,
people try to define them or (worse) try to
shoehorn them into a preconceived notion
of what they want them to be ...?

The problem lies in expectations,
       you said.
People expect too much.

Then you uttered two words
to which I add two more:

"Expect nothing,"
    you said.

"Appreciate everything."

    *   *   *   *
One night

...one day.

...*daybreak*

Every ending
marks
a new beginning.

Welcome to ours.

Wherever it takes us,
      rejoice.

(A Missile in the Mail)

'Couple' defined

"'Thank you' can't adequately say
thanks for what you have done for my
entire being. As I write this,
tears of joy and gratitude spill from
my eyes. Your constant support
has helped me on a daily basis.

"How special you make me feel.
I no longer feel broken. I am whole.
I can love and feel excited
and happy. I can laugh and
my eyes can smile again.

"Thank you for your tenderness,
your closeness, and your sweet
heartfelt words."

    Backatcha, Luv.
    Me, too.
    <RES>

(One more
rather personal
reminder …)

*I love you more
than I have ever loved
anyone else,*

*and more than
anyone else
has ever loved you.*

*And you, my Love,
know who "you" are.*

<RES>

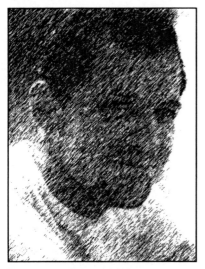

<u>end notes</u>

Selections from (or designated for) other RES works or works in progress:

1. "a warm autumn day on old orchard road" (adapted)
   © *Richard E. Schingoethe (RES)*
2. "someone (not just any …)"
   © *Richard E. Schingoethe (RES)*
3. "from afar" © *Richard E. Schingoethe (RES)*
4. "Life is a Lyric: thoughts on a journey through love and divorce" © *Richard E. Schingoethe (RES)*
5. (As scored) "S & S Suite Mix …I"
   © *Richard E. Schingoethe (RES) and Theodore H. Sieber*
6. "Gifted: a love story in three hearts"
   © *Richard E. Schingoethe (RES)*
7. "Just around the corner" Lyric & Music by
   Richard E. Schingoethe (RES) and Theodore H. Sieber
8. "one day" © *Richard E. Schingoethe (RES)*

LaVergne, TN USA
26 August 2009

155822LV00003B/10/P